Social Work From A Therapeutic Orientation

Social Work From A Therapeutic Orientation

by J. Lea Koretsky

REGENT PRESS
Berkeley, California

Copyright© 2012 by Judy Koretsky

Paperback Version
ISBN 13: 978-1-58790-192-8
ISBN 10: 1-58790-192-7

E-Book Version
ISBN 13: 978-1-58790-193-5
ISBN 10: 1-5890-193-5

Library of Congress Catalog Number: 2012932608

Manufactured in the United States of America
REGENT PRESS
www.regentpress.net
regentpress@mindspring.com

Table of Contents

Introduction / 7

Foreword / 9

Psychological Evaluation / 13

The Laws Governing Child Abuse / 17

The New Psychopathology / 27

Case Management Issues / 35

The Process of Gaining Insight / 89

Literature Review / 95

The Petitions / 111

The Model for the Interviews / 129

Treatment Problems / 139

The Specialized Modalities / 159

Narcissism / 179

Appendixes /

First Interview With Parents / 187

Commonly Asked Questions / 189

Charts / 206

Suggested Reading / 213

Introduction

Insight into one's behavior creates enhanced awareness. Over time increased tolerance to ambivalence produces personal change. This process depends on shifting emphasis from self-negation and a pseudo-self to learning how to respond in ways that do not fuel intolerance, spite or violence to others. People who grow up with abuse eventually stifle their common sense. Abuse may be quite serious from beating up a child and wounding or injuring him; to locking him in a closet for hours or days causing dehydration and terror. Some people develop rage and antipathy while others shut down in a numbness of depression. Children act out often becoming anti-social, criminally prone and combative. As the individual of these families becomes an adult he separates from his inner self.

Social work is a mandated service which modifies living circumstances in order to protect the safety of the child. Its main objective is to produce better decisions in the protective adult and change in the abusive parent through the rendering of therapy, education, treatment and insight into one's own triggers and adaptation to inability to cope. Teaching parents choices for giving children safety within the home environment and in life is the essential outcome.

Foreword

This book comes as a result of over 42,000 face-to-face adult and child interview hours combined in career fields of group work and child abuse investigation and social welfare service from 1986 to 2005. For the recommended treatment discussed here, outcomes were based upon 2,150 adults and 820 children. The system of social work which aims at restoring families to a former optimum level of functioning, spends considerable time monitoring the use of services meant to provide families with alternate information and capable skills to greatly decrease the possibility of risk of detriment to children. I began with a central question – how does change in behavior occur? Issues involved the complexity of risk for which, if the family were to regroup at some point in the future, risk would have to be eliminated, were studied. Issues were defined as consisting of physical abuse, severe neglect, maternal deprivation including depression and schizophrenia, danger including drug and substance abuse, and hostility and humiliation such as is found in molestation.

A second question was asked as to when to bring in independent therapists to produce successful outcomes. The adults received a minimum of twelve hours in the first four weeks prior to a determination being made as to whether to bring in outside therapists to work with family members. Those original twelve hours, each based on a traditional therapy hour, involved assessments of family of origin and extended family for the purposes of establishing safety, setting up contracts, arranging hospitalization, and providing short term, immediate negotiation for parent/teen conflicts, estranged family and custodial parents, teens in trouble with the legal system and frequently combative addicted parties, in addition to the standard orientation required in order to adequately put therapy for the case plan effectively into place.

Individual studies are presented for areas concerned with the efficacy of lesser used modalities, hostile narcissism as a significant cause of perpetration and maternal deprivation as it relates to defensive detachment syndrome. On the objectives of relatedness and relating, the criteria used was derived from my work with group practice – modeling responsiveness, examining situations previously of low tolerance, acknowledging ambivalence, and incorporating structure into personal activities.

Overcoming resistance was determined on one factor of participation – what each person in a family said had to match what both the police report and the victimized child said as to what happened in the critical event of abuse, before re-integration could begin.

Finally satisfactory completion was based upon a change in attitude for which self-insight occurred when objectivity was gained and the parent could accept loss of the previous functioning of the relationship without being defensive. Outcomes included –

> *Substantially decreased risk of detriment*
> *Tolerance for large amounts of anxiety*
> *Development of empathy*
> *Bonding attachment, and*
> *Increased sensitivity for the personal rights of others*

These outcomes were charted on the basis of allegation of child abuse and sex. Lower outcomes were seen in those situations where the adult being treated was unwilling to look at personal issues or held unrealistic objectives despite there being clear alternatives.

The resulting cohesive schedule of family contacts and rationale for marginal compliance, test lab results and clinical methodology was formulated in order to inform the Superior Court Judge as to the child's stability and sensitivities and to establish a thoroughly documented chronology of case work, arranged and supervised visitation between the child or children and the offender, therapy hours with the family and the child, education reports, and any other reports such as psychological and academic evaluations.

Special thanks go to John DiMello, MFC, for his extensive work on modules related to substance misuse and sex molestation for his unique development of treatment and to Dr. Dennis Banks, PhD, for his substance recovery program New Connections in the outpatient milieu. Thanks also go to Dr. John Sutterfield, PhD, Dr. Eliana Gil, PhD, and Dr. Sue Scoff, PhD, of Concord, California and to Diversion 1000 for their work with offenders in the field of exploitation.

December, 2011
Judy Lea Koretsky

Psychological Evaluation

The task of the treating social worker is to assure safety of a child in the home. The job involves implementing a case plan ordered by the Superior Court. This plan lists activities the parent must complete in order to regain custodial control of their child. During the life of the case the social worker must instruct, coach and provide counseling as he or she coordinates and assesses for outcomes. For this social workers must have at their disposal a complex comprehensive psychologically based orientation for usual problems including substance abuse, neglect, cruelty, emotional abuse, molestation, incest, and abandonment. In addition, they must be able to differentiate between unhealthy and crucial and appropriate bonding and attachment between parent and child. The extent of the depression and grief expressed by the child necessarily determines the regrouping of the family. If there is substantial risk to the child, the social worker drafts allegations based upon the evidence which can include fractures, bruises or welts or can include hearsay such as when a child alleges molestation. The social worker must be able to state under what circumstances the child is affected; then must address the conditions which if complied with in a case plan could produce a stable secure home for the particular child. To be able to proceed from allegation to reintegration of the family, the social worker should be steeped in theory, know what treatments work for most adults, and then provide written advisement to the court. This presentation must state the presenting problem and advance wording which informs the judge or commissioner of the continued maladaptive behavior, the current extent of the parent's neglect or detriment, and if needed offer changes to the plan that guides the case.

Foster care is perceived to give the child further psychological remedy. There is ample therapeutic orientation that speaks to the child's emotional needs in various model communities. Under many plans the social worker provides the intervention and thus it is usual and customary for a public servant to provide art therapy, play, complete visitation arrangements, do onsite school observations and a host of other functions.

The schools of psychological thought join as to ways in which individuals undergo healing of overly rigorous or neglectful behaviors to teens and children. Socialization of the parent in the role as limit setter is a subject of discourse of regimen for therapy. Likewise factual information about addiction and resultant abuse discusses the denial system of both the addictive person and those who are dependent on him. Since we already know that denial carries with it a rigid structure intended psychologically to facilitate the family's secrets, we must look to structures where the method of maladaptive coping may have been useful to the family. Rehabilitation often relies on a change in the family system to a structure that empowers each participant's inquiry into self and provides some mirroring of the external world.

Just as a therapy group is governed by increased self awareness of members as they interact, so a family is based upon systems that enhance or contain roles. As family members shed their denial, they begin to inculcate the trust they perceive others respond to them with. As the case progresses to four or five months, the issues that emerge include: emotional boundaries, becoming increasingly open, dealing with personal bugaboos, acknowledging control issues, expressing fears and allowing others to support. Also helping parents develop a personal metaphor gives each child a method for exploring life concerns with a meaningful perspective. Dreams, writing and humor add to dispell the falsely erected barriers meant to achieve control over what might be otherwise painful experiences of youth and adulthood.

The process of discovery of what makes people with similar experience fallback to certain behaviors facilitates an awareness of differences of understanding of experience. This realization as to how each person responds begins to weave an expanded repertoire available to each. A process that gives each person the ability to learn to choose interactions rather than be mysteriously drawn and controlled by them shifts emphasis onto sifting through the process for common ground, evaluating the significance to one's life and over time inculcating what is of value.

From a public welfare stance the aids for recovery include education, therapy groups, individual counseling and social welfare support including counseling. With these aids, the objective of the court is for the abusing or negligent parent to produce insight into behavior such that constructive change is observable. The treating social work practitioner has to instruct the family as outcomes are accomplished what further therapy is designed to provide and a capable working definition as to when and how personal change occurs. The complexity of case management draws upon an essential practicum of awareness as the key to change. Gradual awareness permits the individuals being treated to come into self responsibility such that as one's definition for responsible parenting is advanced so is their ability to tolerate milestones inherent in their child's behaviors.

The Law Governing Child Abuse

The first goal in treatment is to make certain the parent has an adequate understanding of the sustained petition in which the facts of the case are written for the pertinent section of the law that has been adjudicated.

The section of the law regarding dependent children is 300. The selected paragraphs of each law read:

"Any minor who comes within any of the following descriptions is within the jurisdiction of the juvenile court which may adjudge that minor to be a dependent child of the court —

(a) The minor has suffered, or there is a substantial risk that the minor will suffer, serious physical harm inflicted non accidentally upon the minor by the minor's parent or guardian.

(b) The minor has suffered, or there is a substantial risk that the minor will suffer, serious physical harm or illness, as a result of the failure or inability of his or her parent or guardian to adequately supervise or protect the minor, or the willful or negligent failure of the minor from the conduct of the custodian with whom the minor has been left, or by the willful or negligent failure of the parent or guardian to provide the minor with adequate food, clothing, shelter or medical treatment, or by the inability of the parent or guardian to provide regular care for the minor due to the parent's or guardian's mental illness, developmental disability, or substance abuse.

(c) The minor is suffering serious emotional damage, or is at substantial risk of suffering serious emotional damage, evidenced by severe anxiety, depression, withdrawal, or untoward aggressive behavior toward self or others, as a result of the conduct of the parent or providing appropriate care.

(d) The minor has been sexually abused, or there is a substantial risk that the minor will be sexually abused, as defined in Section 11165.1 of the Penal Code, by his or her parent or the guardian or a member of his or her parent or guardian or a member of his or her household, or the parent or guardian has failed to adequately protect the minor from sexual abuse when the parent or guardian knew or reasonably should have known that the minor was in danger of sexual abuse.

(e) The minor is under the age of five and has suffered severe physical abuse by a parent, or any person known by the parent, if the parent knew or reasonably should have known that the person was physically abusing the minor.

(f) The minor's parent or guardian has been convicted of causing the death of another child through abuse or neglect.

(g) The minor has been left without any provision for support; the minor's parent has been incarcerated or institutionalized and cannot arrange for the care of the minor; or a relative or other adult custodian with whom the child resides or has been left is unwilling or unable to provide care or support for the child, the whereabouts of the parent is unknown, and reasonable efforts to locate the parent have been unsuccessful.

(h) The minor has been freed for adoption from one or both parents for 12 months by either relinquishment or termination of parental rights or an adoption petition has not been granted.

(i) The minor has been subjected to an act or acts of cruelty by the parent or guardian or a member of his or her household, or the parent or guardian has failed to adequately protect the minor from an act or acts of cruelty when the parent or guardian knew or reasonably should have known the minor was in danger of being subjected to an act or acts of cruelty.

(j) The minor's sibling has abused or neglected, as defined in subdivision (a), (b), (d), (e) or (i), and there is a substantial risk that the minor will be abused or neglected, as defined in those subdivisions.

"It is the intent of the Legislature in enacting this section to provide maximum protection for children who are currently being physically, sexually, or emotionally abused, being neglected, or being exploited, and to protect children who are at risk of that harm. This protection includes a full array of social and health services to help the child and family and to prevent reabuse of children. That protection shall focus on the preservation of the family whenever possible."

The Rights of Minors / Evidence Code / Section 352
Admitting and Excluding Evidence
Preliminary Determinations

The law on Evidence Code states it is the discretion of the court to exclude evidence. Section 352.1 speaks to Criminal sex acts, as follows:

"In any criminal proceeding under Section 261, Section 264.1, subdivision (d) of Section 286, or subdivision (d) of Section 288a of the Penal Code, or in any criminal proceeding under subdivision (c) of Section 286 or subdivision (c) of Section 288a of the Penal Code in which the defendant is alleged to have compelled the participation of the victim by force, violence, duress, menace, or threat of great bodily harm, the district attorney may, upon written motion with notice to the defendant or the defendant's attorney, if he or she is represented by an attorney, within a reasonable time prior to any hearing, move to exclude from evidence the current address and telephone number of any victim at such hearing."

Other pertinent sections of law address various aspects of the Evidence Code as it may affect the rights of minors.

"405. (a) When the existence of a preliminary fact is disputed, the court shall indicate which party has the burden of producing evidence and the burden of proof on the issue as implied by the rule of law under which the question arises."

"621. (a) Except as provided in subdivision (b), the issue of a wife cohabiting with her husband, who is not impotent or sterile, is conclusively presumed to be a child of the marriage.

(b) Notwithstanding subdivision (a), if the court finds that the conclusions of all experts, as disclosed by the evidence based upon the blood tests performed pursuant to Chapter 2 (commencing with Section 890) of Division 7, are that the husband is not the father of the child, the question of paternity of the husband shall be resolved accordingly."

"802. A witness testifying in the form of an opinion may state on direct examination the reason for his opinion and the matter (including, in the case of an expert, his special knowledge, skill, experience, training, and education) upon which it is based, unless he is precluded by law from using such reasons or matter as a basis for his opinion. The court in its discretion may require that a witness before testifying in the form of an opinion be first examined concerning the matter upon which his opinion is based."

"893. The tests shall be made by experts qualified as examiners of blood types who shall be appointed by the court. "

"912. (a) Except as otherwise provided in this section, the right of any person to claim a privilege provided by Section 954 (lawyer-client privilege), 980 (privilege for confidential marital communication), 994 (physician-patient privilege), 1014 (psychotherapist-patient privilege), 1033 (privilege of penitent), 1034 (privilege of clergyman), or 1035.8 (sexual assault victim-counselor privilege) is waived with respect to a communication protected by such privilege if any holder of the privilege, without coersion, has disclosed to a significant part of the communication or has consented to such disclosure made by anyone. Consent to disclosure is manifested by any statement or other conduct of the holder of the privilege indicating consent to the disclosure, including failure to claim the privilege in any proceeding in which the holder has the legal standing and opportunity to claim the privilege.

(b) Where two or more persons are joint holders of a privilege provided by Section 954, 994, 1014, or 1035.8, a waiver of the right of a particular joint holder of the privilege to claim the privilege does not affect the right of another joint holder to claim the privilege. In the case of the privilege provided by Section 980, a waiver of the right of one spouse to claim the privilege does not affect the right of the other spouse to claim the privilege.

(c) A disclosure that is itself privileged is not a waiver of any privilege.

(d) A disclosure in confidence of a communication that is protected by a privilege provided by Sections 954, 99 4, 1014, or 1035.8, when such disclosure is reasonably necessary for the accomplishment of the purpose for which the lawyer, physician, psychotherapist, or sexual assault counselor was consulted, is not a waiver of the privilege."
"914. (b) No person shall be held in contempt for failure to disclose information claimed to be privileged unless he has failed to comply

with an order of the court that he disclose such information."

"918. (a) (If) the court determines that there is no other feasible means to rule on the validity of such claim other than to require disclosure, the court shall proceed in accordance with subdivision (b).

(b) The court may require to disclose the information in chambers out of the presence of all persons; if the judge determines that the information is privileged, neither he or any other person may ever disclose, without consent of the person authorized to permit disclosure."

"1035.4. The court may compel disclosure of information received by the sexual assault counselor which constitutes relevant evidence of the facts and circumstances involving an alleged sexual assault."

The Evidence Code as to the Child pertains predominantly to admissability of tests, paternity, physical abuse and torture, sexual assault and domestic violence.

Exceptions for disclosure:

A public officer or services specialist or social work professional, licensed as a therapist or psychologist, who may be treating the victim is not regarded as a holder of the privilege.

A victim of domestic violence has a privilege to refuse to disclose and to prevent another from disclosing.

Hearsay Evidence

The hearsay law addresses admissibility of certain out-of-court statements of minors under the age of 12, as for a statement included in a written report of a law enforcement official or an employee of a county welfare department. The statement was made by a minor alleging to be a victim of sexual abuse. The statement was made prior to the defendant's confession. There are no significant inconsistencies that would render the statement inadmissible. The minor is unavailable to be found or refuses to testify.

Areas of Practiced Law as Regards Child Abuse
The areas of law that pertain to the rights of children are listed in an index titled CHILD, Children and Minors. These include but are not limited to:

Abandonment, desertion
Abduction
Arrest, notice to parents
Autopsies
Community treatment facility
Confidentiality
Contracts
Costs, medical costs
Custody proceedings
Domestic violence
Drug addicts
Evidence
Federal aid
Foster homes
Funds
Guardian ad litem
Hearsay evidence
Hospital reports
Information disclosure
Juvenile delinquents
Libel and slander
Licenses and permits
Medical care
Mental health
Multidisciplinary disclosure
Notice

Parole and probation
Records
Refusal to participate
Reports
Residential shelter services
Schools
Temporary custody
Training and prevention
Trust funds
Unlawful corporal punishment
Visitation, best interests of the child
Welfare services
Witnesses
Adoption of children
Adult status, emancipation
AIDS
Anesthetic, consent
Application for driver's license
Paternity
Birth certificates
Blood tests
Change of residence
Citation for misdemeanor offenses
Privileged information
Conservatorship
Probate proceedings
Real estate
Statutory authority
Control of child's property
Child beating
Churches, controlled substances
Defacing property
Degrading or immoral practices
Film, sexual exploitation
Gangs
High schools, controlled substances
Lewdness and obscenity

Oral copulation
Crippled children
Cultural child-rearing practices
Deprivation
Grandparents, visitation
Presumed father
Damages, shoplifting
Deaf and mute persons
Developmentally disabled persons
Education
Genetic defects
Handicapped children
Heirs
Homeless youth
Illegitimate children
Indian child custody
Interstate compact on juveniles
Married minors
Names
Payment of wages
Privileges and immunities
Runaway youth
Tests
Transcripts
Videotapes
Wards of court
Xrays

The law makes no legally binding designations to prevent adult behavior. It only has authority to protect the minor child.

The New Psychopathology

By the early 1970s psychological public policy redefined the term psychopathology in social work to replace the outmoded term sociopathy with its emphasis on child and adolescent psychopharmacology for children suffering from attention deficit hyperactivity disorder, oppositional defiance, bipolar syndrome and depression, anxiety, conduct disorder, gender identity disorder in children, sleep terror disorder and autism spectrum disorders. Within a broader, more egalitarian definition of child and adolescent psychopathy arose the ideas of child abuse and the family system with new awareness of domestic violence and chemical dependency as the impact of these affects the child with endangerment or risk of detriment inside the home. With the advent of child abuse referral networks, removal of children from threat and placement in foster care, the child welfare system had unburdened anti-social adolescents to specialized treatment facilities while multi-tasking out incorrigible youth, teen runaways and teens with special aptitude skills as distinct from the physically abused child, the sexually abused youngster and the neglected pre-adolescent who had no supervision by an adult. This expansion of service added to the predominant physician service which placed a bipolar or conduct disordered adolescent in a hospital locked ward or at a physician-run boy's ranch. Today, when a child is taken from a custodial parent, the police write a removal order permitting the child to stay overnight or over a weekend until the Superior Court judge can extend the placement. No longer a physician decision, the system for child abuse is adjudicated by a juvenile court judge and all child abuse matters segregated from the criminal judicial court process for either child or adult in probation. Thus, management of adolescent psychopaths is curtailed to institutions and agencies where the adolescent attends school at the treatment facility where the teen also receives medication for anxiety, individual and group therapy four times a week, stabilization off drugs or alcohol, and education in self-management and electives.

Managing risk of threat to the child occurs in the court before a Judge in three to eight separate hearings, the first two two weeks apart, each one thereafter at six month intervals. Depending upon the Judge's order for placement in the home or in foster care or group home, the child may reside at home with certain restrictions imposed or will live in someone else's care. The social worker has the responsibility to make certain the child is safe; to assure this, the social worker is expected to visit the child for an in-person interview of one hour minimum each month preferably in the residence with the custodial parent or foster parent.

The balance between the clinical social management professional and the Court has for this reason taken on a reciprocity which may never have been intended. The more capable social worker has clinical training and possibly expertise in making fundamental diagnostic evaluations. For the basic training they receive they are expected to state by virtue of observation and written materials in the case file the severity of detriment to the child as well as to any other child who might enter the home. The professional who engages in this profession must be fully able to correctly identify the client's severe behavior and consistently treat it, even while that individual is treated by a therapist. Because interns are widely used, the degree of expertise is understandably small. The treating social worker must have at their disposal a complex comprehensive psychologically based orientation for these usual problems — substance abuse, neglect, personality disorders, emotional abuse, molestation, incest, and abandonment. In addition, they must be able to demonstrate in spite of negative or positive testing the crucial and appropriate bonding and attachment between parent and child. Likewise for the teen ward of the court there must be some discussion as to psychological precursors that no matter whether treatment could be possible the subjective abuse is determined to be already malicious or detrimental. The social worker needs to enter the judicial arena able to describe the substantiated allegations as the parent's behaviors apply and demonstrate the impact on the child.

All capabilities are predicated upon judicial orders. These orders must be obtained in the specified time frames. Referrals are either deemed to be immediate or ten day status. An immediate referral will be assigned for immediate investigation and filing. The investigation may involve talking to the child; if he has any injury, he must be detained.

24 hours – the filing of the petition.

Two work days – filing for jurisdiction, that is, the injury occurred in the county in which the child resides.

Two weeks – filing for disposition, asking the Judge to award Dependency under W&I Code 300.

Once a referral has been investigated and allegations substantiated under a 300 section, the parents from whom the child is removed are ordered to complete a case plan in order to reunite with their child. This case plan usually consists of three or four requirements but has been known to contain as many as ten required items. Usually requirements include counseling for the child by therapist approved by social services for individual weekly sessions for a minimum of one hour each; conjoint sessions between any dyad or entire family consisting at discretion of family psychotherapist parent and spouse, parent and child, children together or family together; residential or outpatient rehabilitation; substance abuse testing by random or weekly or daily method with negative results; and arranged supervised or unsupervised visitation between parent and child.

ChangingMaladaptive Behavior

The essential task for any case plan lies with the parent who has changed his behavior in a fundamental manner such that the possibility of reoffense is highly unlikely. He has to show that he has thought a good deal about the issues of the allegations and has changed his thinking about the circumstance. He must also exhibit empathy for the child and is deemed capable by the victimized child of rendering an apology in a session with the child and therapist. This process takes a year – six or seven months to establish raporte. Once positive esteem is generated, the therapeutic intervention may take one to two years to resolve the presenting problem. To begin this process the parent has to describe the incident that led to the filing of the petition. It may be he took an argument outside into the street and then punched his wife when she followed. Making changes in behavior requires long hours of listening without forming an opinion. The social worker and possibly a therapist helps him connect his emotional response to its actual stressor if he experiences sadness, loss, or intolerance. For him to have successfully worked through his overload of stress or guilt or defiance may necessitate him talking about his job for several months. It may require that he look at his behaviors in the presence of his family. He may have to stop threatening to make someone pay. He has to ask what he does that scares the child. Is it coercive in nature? Does he sleep sitting up in a chair in the hall with a loaded rifle on his lap? Does he punch his fist into walls when he feels intolerant?

Denial is often the first stage of resistance. Many families are resistant to change. They view the needed alternate course of action as an intrusion into their lives. Some view the case plan requirements as devaluing or consuming too much time. They feel that taking a psychosocial evaluation from a team of psychotherapists, substance testing, weekly individual and family counseling consisting of child sand play, diversion for domestic abuse and a twelve-week parenting class as too demanding, finger pointing, and ' wanting their entire life.' For some parents, talking about intimate details seems intrusive. Often having to acknowledge that an essential betrayal has occurred and produced mistrust, bred ill will, and removed primary affection is painful to realize. Some examples include fondling a step-daughter or walking into the shower with her while she is showering; locking a young child into a closet for days instead of baby-sitting; feeding a baby poison meant to subdue its cries; arm wrestling and thereby causing a sprain or splint; or placing a child's arms or legs in restraints. However, once the risk to the child has been discussed, it is this process of exploring what happened that permits early awareness of the limitations of the spousal relationship, allowing for openness to begin to replace the secretive denial in the family that all is well.

Personal change is governed by increased self awarenes which occurs over time as the individual becomes gradually fluent at therapy. It is the result of practicing new behaviors both through individual psychotherapy and group work. As new skills are tried, they eventually become more adaptable. These skills include learning to tolerate differences of opinion, waiting a week before acting on a decision, adjusting to ambivalence - not knowing what one thinks about something - and deciding not to try to control another person's responses. The group is a clear-seeking method to adopt new behaviors in a safe setting while exploring the aspects of one's life that have rigidly held a sense of fragile Self in place. Understanding this rigidity becomes prominent when conflict arises. Conflict after all challenges one's ability to be flexible. In the case plan personal change is essential. The parent is charged with creating a safer home; to do this, he or she must thoughtfully utilize what is learned in class and counseling in order to provide the child with constructive guidance.

Because insight into one's own behavior is crucial to the

recovery process, the treating practitioner must already have an awareness of what therapy is designed to accomplish and demonstrate a capable working definition as to when and how personal change occurs. The complexity of case management necessarily draws upon an essential practicum of awareness as the key to change. Gradual awareness permits the individuals being treated to come into self responsibility such that as one's definition for responsible parenting is advanced so is their ability to tolerate milestones inherent in their child's behaviors. For this reason group work gives each individual a mirror to their behavior, aids in facilitating the parenting style outside oneself, and provides for seeking support in order to work through various typically held problems. Individual work creates a basis upon which to search for personal meaning. In doing so the individual begins with a series of objectives so that a finding for permanence may be made, as long as the parent can reasonably show they have gained by an improved understanding of their child's needs.

Koretsky introduces a group process that removes the stigma of authoritarian control from the therapist and instead sets all interactions into a group concept allowing each person to sample what they will. This process gives each person what is of value.

Foster care gives the child further psychological remedy. These living environments provide a physically and psychologically safe residence. Many caretakers were parents themselves with a nursing background and provide art therapy, sand tray, safe play with another child and make and supervise visitation arrangements. When they keep teenagers, they take them to soccer or baseball, attend ballet, go to movies and prepare them for college. For additional support they bring them to Alateen, Alanon, or Alcoholics Anonymous which helps teens become better adjusted socially.

In order to be able to proceed from admitting the truth inherent in the allegations of the petition, the social worker has to be able to assure the Court what insights the parents have had. The social worker has to list the services of the case plan that the parents have attended and write a summary with the opinions of both each parent and each therapist. For substance abuse residential rehabilitation a parent who was a former drug addict has to say how much of the drug they consumed as well as the frequency. For example he has to acknowledge he snorted a bag a day and when he couldn't afford it, he purchased "snot" or "ice" which are both forms of methamphetamine. He has to test weekly with negative results every test. Then he has to describe his life without the drug. He may be calm; he may remember. When he visits with his son, he may be able now to sit for a few hours and draw pictures and build a sandcastle. He can look back at his past behavior and understand and describe that he was excessively harsh. He lacked any ability to know his own limits. He will say, A keen mind is a clean mind. As he begins to walk the walk, he will increase in coping and will be willing to treat others with a seeking mind.

Case Management Issues

Case A

03-02-97 Before my first session at the Agency clinic with the biological parents of S. I discussed with the psychologist her report in my file. I ascertained that I received it with the case record. She stated she met with the family once, then with the parents twice and the child for a half hour. The family sat as follows, father, mother, child. The allegation is that a family friend staying over awakened in the night, found the child watching TV in her bed, lay on the bed with her, fell asleep and at some point after she fell asleep she woke up to his rubbing his penis against her leg. She is eight.

The family seems forthright. I asked how they were referred. The father said they went to see the psychologist after the principal at the girl's school spoke to him and his wife at his office. The father did all the talking with his wife and child sitting silent. He said he works at a law firm in the city. His net pay is $60,000 a year. Although he is not rich he sends his daughter to a Christian school. The male in question is an associate whom he has known about twenty years. He was in college with this friend. His wife works at the college he attended for twenty-five years netting about $25,000 a year.

I asked the girl to wait in the hall while I met with her parents. I gave them a contract for contact, which he agreed to and signed. I said I would see the girl at a separate time weekly. This was fine. I said they needed to arrange a sitter and gave them a list of names.

I spoke to the parents for about forty minutes. The wife said she feels the situation is sad because he is a family friend but she trusts her daughter. Her plan is to supervise more cautiously. She said her husband is fairly liberal with his friends. I asked if he believed his daughter, he said she is too young to tell a lie.

I obtained a marital history. He grew up locally and his wife is from out of the area. They fell in love and dated a few months before they got married at the justice of the peace. They were married two years when she discovered she was pregnant. She loves her husband very much and thinks they can get back to being a family right away.

I then met with the girl. I asked whether she feels safe in her family home. She said she does if her dad's friend does not return. I asked whether what happened scared her. She said not at first. She said when she saw his eyes were closed she did not feel she could ask him to leave. She said since she told her mother she feels she is okay. Her mother has asked her to tell her everything that is not okay.

03-02-97 I called the child's therapist at school. She is a psychologist I am familiar with. She said the girl told another student about the incident who told the school nurse. A conference was held during which the principal asked both parents to come to meet with him. During the meeting the father became angered and told the school to stay out of his business. The principal said a referral was made for a psychological evaluation for the parents. The child's therapist said she sees the girl weekly and she has her do play therapy. There seems to be no unusual ideation.

03-07-97 I met with the child who said her mother told her she and her father are separating temporarily. I asked what she thought the reason might be. She said her parents were arguing about the family friend after her mother made a call to the man's brother. The child said now she wished she hadn't said anything.

I met with the mother who came without the father. The mother said I might as well know the father is not her child's real father. The male's brother is the real father. She has had no contact with this male since she married her husband. She said her husband thinks his friend is the natural father and accused his wife of tricking him into marriage. He demanded to know. She said she does not want to expose her child to any stress.

03-14-97 I met with mother for the first half hour session. Mother stated her husband has cut off all financial support and has moved into a hotel. She has begun looking for a job with more flexible hours. She cannot afford daycare so she has enrolled her child in an after school arts program at the child's school. She is very upset about the way this has evolved. She feels her husband has done this to provoke her into telling him who the father is. She says he is not the father. She won't say who is.

I discussed with her the ramifications of how this may affect her legal rights as to longterm custody. I said I was obligated to declare an absent father. I asked whether he had ever provided any financial support. She said he offered his name on the birth certificate and wanted to pay for health care but she refused. She got a job. He bought her a house.

03-14-97 I contacted the official record for a deed on her house. The deed is in her name.

I drafted a petition declaring an absent father under a 300(g) alleging abandonment. Took it to the County Recorder. I notified parent of morning hearing. She cannot be present.

03-15-97 I appeared in court to enter petition. I requested counsel for mother and absent father. Attorneys assigned. Jurisdiction set for two days.

I went to school to obtain records on child and met with school psychologist who believes child is becoming somewhat withdrawn. I met with child, child was happy to see me. I asked how things are at home. Child said her mother was crying about her job. She said her dad went on a business trip. She had a bad dream. I ascertained child wants to stay at home with her mom.

03-17-07 Juris. Attorneys filed for disclosure. Absent father in court. He gave his name and address, his social security and birth date. He told the court he wanted to be tested for paternity. Court referred. Judge put over hearing until mother can appear.

03-21-07 I met with mother and S. Mother said S. is having trouble sleeping. She wakes up about 3am crying. Mother brings her to her bed and holds her until she falls asleep. Tells S. she loves her. In the morning she fixes her breakfast, they review her homework and then she drives S to school. She described a new schedule she has for S. She picks her up after school all days but one when an older female comes to after-school program for arts. She picks up two of S. female peers who reside in neighborhood. She fixes a snack for the three girls, then has them play in living room and backyard until dinner. I asked S. about these friends. They are girls who attend her school but come home two hours earlier. She knows everything about them. One girl has no father. That girl lives with her mother and grandmother. I asked S. how she likes this new schedule. She said she likes it better than before. She is not so lonely.

03-22-97 Juris. Mother asked for trial requesting absent's parental rights be terminated and no plan for services be offered him. Contested disposition set for two weeks. Paternity test ordered.

I met with mother privately. I spoke to her about the objectives of a trial, that she might have to take S. for a blood test, and if the test proved paternity absent would be granted a plan. She said this was the male who molested S. She felt she was being given a conflicting message. I asked what happened to the brother. She said she was feeling defensive and lied. She said everyone in his family is crazy, they are obsessed with making money. I inquired whether she received any financial assistance from him. She said no, she had done everything she possibly could to get away from him. She was no longer tied to him at all. She said she was transferring to another office and would start in a week. He knew her associates where she was working.

I then asked her attorney if he needed information. He said he would send his secretary to obtain discovery. He wanted to know if we would want visitation for absent father. I told him the agency would need to see longterm therapy first since it was he who abused the child.

That afternoon I met with the consultant psychologist for the agency at the agency's request. He recommends a formal therapist for S. and will assign her to his staff. The psychologist will assess for distress, eneuresis, thumb sucking, inappropriate peer play, continued night problems, etc. The treating psychologist can then testify in court as to sustained trauma and make recommendations as to frequency of visitation.

03-29-07 I met with S. and her mother. I asked S. to select a toy she thought her mother would enjoy. S. went to the shelf with the toys and took a Sesame character puppet and handed it to her mom. I asked S. to tell her mom a story about the toy. S. said, "This is Fred. He is a bad boy even though he acts nice most of the time. He should not be left alone with good children."

I agreed with her saying, "You're right. Fred was a bad boy. He was not behaving appropriately with you. I know you thought you could trust him and I don't think you can. I agree he should not be alone with children."

I asked her mother to respond to her. Her mother said, "I love you with all my heart. I am angry he hurt you the way he did. He should have stayed in the living room and not come into your bedroom."

"I would like to talk to S. Is it alright with you if your mother takes Fred into the waiting room while I talk to you?"

S. gave a nod, but seemed unhappy.

I asked, "Are you upset at Fred?"

S. seized Fred and yelled, "You're the worst thing that has ever happened to me! How could I let you into my house?"

"Did you hear your mother say that?"

S. nodded. "I could hear her through the TV."

"What did you think when you heard your mother say that?"

"Daddy called. I answered the phone. He said he was coming over this weekend to take me to the zoo."

"You must miss him alot. This has to be hard for you to have your father on a business trip."

"I heard Mommy say - how dare you call at this late hour. It wasn't real late, only 8:30. I had taken my bath, brushed my hair and kissed Mommy goodnight when the phone rang."

I said to her mother, "What upset you?"

Her mother looked uncomfortable. "Her father knows I'm getting her ready for bed. Usually I read to her. His call made her want to stay up."

"It's a hard time right now. It sounds like Daddy won't be home for a while but he'll see you this weekend."

"I don't want him to get mad."

"What could he get mad about?"

"He wants Mommy to put a lock on my door. Mommy said she refused."

Her mother said, "I want you to feel safe. I don't want you to feel that a lock is needed. Bad Fred isn't coming to the house ever again."

"Is dad?"

I asked S., "What is your dad's relationship to Fred?"

"Dad drives to work with Fred."

"Maybe your dad can get his own car."

Her mother said, "Fred and dad work at the same place. Fred got dad that job."

"I'm wondering if I can talk to you, S."

"That would be alright."

Her mother left the room. I said to S. "You are not to blame for what Fred did to you. Do you know that?"

"My mom told me that."

"Good. It's important to me that you know you have every right to feel safe. Do you think it would help if you change your room so that you can sleep?"

S. looked sad. "Maybe."

"Alright, this is hard because you grew up in that room. It is part of you. Your memory is telling you something scary happened there."

"A new bed might be good."

"I'm going to suggest that to your mom. I think your mom should take you for a new bed."

"I hadn't thought of that. Do you think Fred was drunk?"

"I'm not sure. I'll have to ask your mother."

"Fred comes over when Daddy wants to drink."

A child may express loyalty at this early stage of therapy to make certain her mother isn't going to leave her too. I have to assume

S. may not be able to call her dad on a regular basis. The child wants to talk about some aspect of her parents' friendship with Fred and is unsure how to do this without violating unspoken understandings that have been operating for this family.

I met with the mother briefly. I asked her about buying S. a new bed and looking through a catalog to agree on which one. I then asked about S.'s perception that Fred has a necessary relationship to her father. The mother said the two work for the same firm and commute together. She said Fred used to bring over wine for dinner and the two would spend the evening talking business. I asked her what she meant by "the whole family is crazy." She said Fred made a killing on children's puzzle games. The family brainstorms on ideas and then Fred creates games.

04-03-07 Contested review. Findings: two hour trial summed up as follows: paternity test positive, father alleged. Allegation sustained. No reunification. Normalization case plan ordered. Goals of therapy to determine if father can become safely empathic and appropriate. No visitation during first year until therapist approves contact. Case plan as to mother to remain as is. Visitation with presumed father must be supervised and can occur in family home. Restraining order for alleged father to stay away from family home, child's school, all friends, therapy.

04-05-07 I met with S.'s mother alone. S. is with babysitter this afternoon. The mother and I discussed the court hearing. She is feeling more supported by the court. She feels she has more control now. She has felt in limbo for weeks. She said she called her mother to determine if she can keep S. for a month while she gets her life straightened out. We discussed this. Is this a good idea at this time? She feels S. will be fine at her mother's and it will give S. some psychological space from her. Her mother has a cabin at a lake.

I felt the mother was somewhat evasive. Clearly she wants time to herself; she's feeling burnt out over the ordeal. She's ambivalent about her husband whom she knows has daily contact with Fred, but the roles are reversed and she believes her husband may withdraw from her and S. while sticking around Fred more. That's how he is. When stressed he spends lots of time at Fred's. She is certain he still doesn't know anything about Fred being S.'s dad. She doesn't think Fred will say anything to him for awhile. Fred likes to keep secrets.

I asked her, what about wanting to get as far away from Fred as possible. She meant financially. She doesn't want him to control her monetarily. She says he has a habit of wanting too much control. When she met him he would lock her inside his house so she was unable to leave before he returned. When he learned she was pregnant by him he wouldn't permit her to leave the house at all. She had to wait for him to go to work, then climbed over the fence to get out and left. She described Fred as combative, jealous, generally blaming.

Fred as described as having a personality disorder that is not managed and thus he is detrimental to the well being of intimates.

04-12-07 I met with S. alone for an hour. I asked how things are going. S. said she went to her grandmother's for a week. She slept really well, went with her grandmother to work, saw two movies. Fred's brother came to take her home. S. said he's her mother's favorite friend. I asked if he has been to the home, S. said no. Her father doesn't like him. He says Fred's brother is poor. I talked to S. about coming home. That was nice. Her mother got her a new bedroom set. It consists of a bed, a desk, a set of drawers and the TV has been moved out of her room into a den.

04-12-07 I met for consultation with a youth services psychotherapist regarding S. I described S.'s awakings at night, her perceptions of Fred, her ability to openly talk about these, and the issue as to transportation and visitation. I was advised, transportation only by mother.

I arranged a time to meet with mother and her mother.

04-13-07 I met with mother at grandmother's home early evening. We discussed how S.'s visit went. Both women felt it was good for S. I asked if this could occur monthly. They would like to do that. I asked mother if she could bring and pick up S. She can. Grandmother said Fred's brother is a friend. I said I had to research this further but for the time being he could not see S. alone. Grandmother wanted to know why. We discussed S. difficulty sleeping and her trust, knowing there are family secrets but not knowing what they are.

They debated if S. ought to be told who her father is. I said I might have to place her in a protective home. The mother says she wants Jim involved because otherwise Fred just shows up. Jim talks to Fred and keeps him manageable. We discussed the problem of recurring fears for a child. I complimented mother for psychologically reassuring S. She said it was her mother's idea.

"Sometimes," I began, with every effort to be educational, "we tell ourselves that trauma goes away when the perpetrator is gone, but for S. she sees indicators of a continued relationship. When this occurs most people react instead of telling themselves they are not helpless. You, Mom, are fearful of Fred yourself. Jim appears to be a good influence for you."

"Yes," the mother said, "I've known Fred a long time. Eventually he does crazy things."

Grandmother said, "He already wanted to take S. to her first prom when she turns 12. My daughter said absolutely not and asked Jim. It was Jim who talked to Fred. Fred, we thought, backed down."

"It's not as though I've kept secrets. I told my husband there was another man before I met him, but he thinks Fred introduced us. At the time I thought getting to know Peter was a good way of getting rid of Fred."

"How is Jim related to you?"

Grandmother said, "He is my stepson. I married Fred's stepfather. Technically I am not related to Fred. My daughter has known Fred since she was six. I told myself after Jim's dad passed, I would be there for him. As a result we are quite close."

"That's a positive response. Jim is lucky. Fred appears to have behaviors that concern me. He cannot know how S. is doing. I wonder whether you could suggest a way to deal with this. What do you think about Fred?"

"He is troubled. He worries my daughter may cut him out of the family."

"Is he close to you?"

"No, his primary friend is the husband. Fred is not one to let people go."

"Do you find his need a problem?"

"No, I don't allow Jim here. He comes to visit at my cabin."

The view for management in this family derives from a belief that one's house is one's castle. It is the husband who has moved out, presumably to keep Fred away from the child he considers his. Even though the child was born after the parents married, the problem is Fred's paternity test was positive for paternity. In addition, although mother changed her name and purchased the house, the house originally belonged to Fred who gave it to the parents for support of the child.

"Is the husband on S.'s birth certificate?"

The mother said, "I wrote that the father was unknown. The nurse at the hospital said my husband did not test for paternity."

Because the husband did not test as being the father, his name was withheld, and the law does not view him as a biological father. This is one of the essential laws that greatly complicate the judicial process governing what must occur.

04-19-07 I met with the husband and S. Their interaction was characterized by warm empathy, genuine communication, honest feedback. S. told her dad she misses him, to which he responded with tears. He called her his "little penguin." He said he thinks about how she's doing but because he has to work closely with Fred for his job, he is temporarily living out of the home until Fred is better. He said Fred is in therapy because he did a bad thing to her. He wants to take her places only when Fred has to be out of town. Her mother, dad says, is his life.

"That's not fair," S. said. "I should be able to live with you. Why can't you get another job?"

Father was silent, debating what to say.

I asked, "Do you want to tell me what keeps you at your job?"

He answered, couching his remarks. "I'm the only person the contract agrees to have work there because of what I know."

"Can you look for another job?"

"I have been trying, but I don't feel that would necessarily be a good idea, at least not right away."

"Will you reassure your daughter?"

He took a deep breath. "Honey, my job is also very important to me. Sometimes life forces us to make decisions we'd rather not make."

I said, "That's a daddy's problem. Not all parents have that option. It's hard to think about, isn't it?"

S. said, "Yes. I don't like Fred anymore."

The father said, rather uncomfortably, "I like him because he helps me."

I swiftly came to S.'s defense. I said, "Fred violated S.'s trust. He made an inappropriate advance to her."

He said, "I asked my wife what happened. She told me something. I can't see him doing what my wife said."

"What did she say?"

"She said he rubbed himself against her."

"Yes," I said, "that's what happened."

"My wife told me to get out. That's why I'm out."

"Did you think what he did was alright?"

"Well, no, but it isn't like it's kissing or something much worse."

I said to S. "I have to ask your dad to have supervised visits from now on. To do this, I must give the judge an immediate report as to our discussion here."

"I could shut you down if I wanted."

"I need for you to step into the hall, please."

He turned to his daughter and placed what was intended to be a reassuring touch to her hand.

I said, "She's not the adult here. You are. She probably wants to know why you continue to have a friendship with him."

"Because if I don't he said he will prevent me from working elsewhere. I can't afford that. I want to be the one who puts a roof over your head. I want you to know I love you. I want you to be your special little self," and he broke into a sob.

04-20-07 Judge ordered all family to the afternoon hearing. The review commenced at 3pm, when all parties had arrived. The child's psychologist has recommended two visits with presumed father per month if child wants and these should occur either at grandmother's or at agency. The judge admonished the fathers. He told them they can both lose parental rights. He approved visitation as to grandmother with the proviso only she transport. No one to discuss any aspect of case except with agency. Stay away orders were updated. Child minor to receive therapy twice a week, therapy to include play therapy. No contact presumed father to alleged except at work.

I met briefly with each adult after hearing. I told mother she has to at some point counsel the minor as to what she wants to keep in place for her protection.

I met with husband and told him he needs to put separation between him and Fred in a tangible way.

I met with Fred and said his case plan objectives are as follows:

He must enter insight therapy with licensed therapist who has at least two years in child abuse counseling, can have been a previous social worker; he has to demonstrate full responsibility for his inappropriate behavior to S., get sober, and then he has to change his behavior and have an apology session. There will be no contact until that occurs. If after that occurs he reoffends any child, he will lose parental rights and get arrested and it will stay on his record.

04-21-07 I went to S.'s school to see S. I asked her previous psychologist to join us. We were given the principal's office in which to meet. I asked S. how she was doing. She said she hit another child on the playground. I asked how that came about.

"The kid said they knew my parents were divorced."

Her psychologist said, "S. was very upset after this occurred. She was crying. I called her mother who came and got her. We talked about the incident. I advised her to take her to her counselor and suggested she call you."

I explained that her father has not severed the friendship with the abuser. Their father/child relationship is newly affected. I thought S. should be seen daily for school counseling and her teachers to be alerted to any distress she may begin to have. I asked S. about her perceptions of yesterday's discussion. She said she didn't think it was fair that she couldn't concentrate.

The interrelationship between therapists, agency and school is complex although necessary. They hold a joint responsibility to make certain the child does not show further signs of fragmentation. The child has suffered loss of attachment, she will begin to undergo grief and anger, remorse will emerge possibly in the forms of anger, feelings of an essential rejection, possibly a belief that she is overwhelmed.

I then met with S. alone. I asked how she likes her other therapist. She likes her therapist but says she is being treated as a child. All they do is color and play with toys. Her therapist asked her yesterday whether she wanted to visit her grandmother. She said her father came to take her out but she told her mother she didn't want to go with him. I said it could be she is angrier than she expected to be. I said her future visits with her dad were cut to twice a month, but only if she wants to see him, and will be at her grandmother's or here. She said she would like them at her grandmother's.

04-28-07 I saw the mother at her home. The house is a small two bedroom, clean, artistic with nice furniture, antique cabinets and tables, the kitchen was modernized with glass cabinets, formica, overlooking a small patio. She took me to see S. in her room. It is very pretty, lots of loving gestures, books, toys, a small desk, a large closet filled with pretty clothing. She picked out her favorite dresses. Her grandmother takes her to church whenever she goes there. GM said father will join them. S. is in a special class at school. She had to memorize a poem and say it from memory to her class and she has an hour of track and runs. She said she thinks fine again.

I talked to the mother in the living room. I asked what S.'s therapist tells her about S. The mother said she meets with Dr. C for ten minutes each session. Dr. C says S. suffers from post traumatic stress syndrome related to child abuse by a person other than the family. Dr. C has advised her to set S. up for choral group which she plans to have her mother do. Dr. C also suggests private junior high school which she will talk to her husband about.

I asked about her own therapy. She sees a therapist for a half hour every week during which she reports on a parenting class, contact with S.'s school and arrangements for visitation with her husband. The remainder of time, about 20 minutes, is spent talking about S.'s trauma. Her psychotherapist wants her to first see things from S.'s viewpoint. Once she is able to discuss her thoughts about the molest, he will extend the time to forty minutes. I asked if it is useful. She says she answers his questions but doesn't know what he wants from her. She asks him for examples but he doesn't say much.

I asked if she knows anyone who has ever done therapy. She said no, it's for sick people. I asked her if that is her mother's attitude. She doesn't know. She hasn't talked with her mother. I then asked what her upbringing consisted of. She is a non practicing Christian. Her mother works for a group of lawyers, her father while he was living was a corporate lawyer. She is an only child of his and has a stepbrother Jim. Jim's father was a soft spoken minister who was very tolerant. He took them in after her dad passed. Her dad was in his 70s, when her mother was 30. She regarded her parents' relationship as very funny, loving, exciting, whereas her stepfather was more mild by nature, helpful without being gregarious. She got close to Jim first, and he has proved to remain a longterm friend. Jim in some way replaced her dad. Because of this, she always goes to him to sort out her conflicts.

I asked her what he has told her about Fred. Jim thought he should have been hospitalized permanently. Jim believes he has problems relating emotionally. Around women he is awkward, drinks, becomes demanding, but for a much younger person he is seductive, although untruthful even though he doesn't say much. Jim is of the opinion he should marry her and reside in Arizona with his aunt. I asked what she knows about this person. She met her a few times. She runs a typing service for several groups of lawyers. S.'s mother believes running to the southwest would not be helpful for S. I wanted to know if Fred would have any way to learn. She shut down, today her face was impassive. I asked what happened, and she replied she felt criticized.

I said, "Fred has enormous control over this family."

"Tell me about it."

"Any possibility he will not agree to your taking your daughter outside the state?"

"Try the city, try the neighborhood."

"What did he do after you escaped his yard?"

"He came to a shelter, left his radio in his car on, slammed his fist on the door. I was thrown out."

"Did you call the police?"

"No, I called my mother."

"So he wants you to stay a little girl."

"I couldn't call the cops. He would've returned to make trouble. I've been through that."

"What do you tell Jim?"

"That I'm not as happy as I was but at least I have my freedom. That my mother still wants to cosign for us, that I was told by a coworker I don't make the grade. Just things."

"Do you know what he says to Fred?"

"Sometimes. He says we're down on our luck, that the house is too small, S. is growing up fast."

"S. is too young to be on her own. She has to stay at least until age 18. S. sometimes has to say what she thinks should have occurred ---"

"No," she interrupted, "that's her father. Everyone has to do that."

"Can you explain that?"

She shifted her position. "He never breaks off a relationship. He always keeps secrets. He thinks what happened to S. did not involve him. That's what he's made of. He compartmentalizes."

"S. overheard an outburst to the effect of, Fred, you are the worst thing that ever happened to me. What is that?"

"I think Fred knew what he was doing. He said he was drunk. I think even if he was drunk he did not have to do it."

I waited.

"What was the question again?"

"The outburst."

"Oh, right. I think he thought he would do the same thing with her. He did that to me. I had asked S. what he did. It's exactly the same. I don't want her to wind up in his dungeon."

"Were you 11?"

"No, I was 16."

"That's a big difference. At 16 if you aren't related, that could be consentual."

"He's my cousin."

"That's consentual. This is not because she is a child."

"Now you know."

"I'd like you to discusss with your therapist this issue. My impression is that you will protect up to a certain age and then in some sense release her psychologically. What do you think?"

"I think I'd like my husband home. He works with Fred, not for him. I can take him to work and S. to school. There's no need to drag this out. I could put a lock on her door but we're not the problem. We just won't allow her to have Fred come over. Then the matter is closed."

"What about Jim? He gives your information to Fred."

"I can't be fixed. What's done is done."

"I think now that you are willing to discuss the issues, you can look at them in therapy and I will monitor for six months. If S. continues to be stable, then I will try to recommend permanent custody to you with no contact to Fred for S. But typically we hold to these cases a year."

My sense of the mother is she is still not being forthright. I have obtained birth certificates for all, I have asked for a search for any psychiatric records for Fred. My concern is why the family does not isolate from Fred by redefining their social support and why they don't bring other adults into their home. My belief is because mother has been dependent on Fred for all emotional support, she does not think to provide a wider support network.

The federal law which governs child abuse says every effort has to be given a biological parent the opportunity for reconciliation. If anything happens to the mother in the future, the agency will reopen the case and contact the other parent that has paternity proven. For reunification of any type to occur the biological parent if he has a problem that prohibits contact or places restrictions on contact, he must be given time and services to fix his problem. Different counties draw on different interpretations. In California, Lake County has a very small budget and they have five social workers to handle everything as opposed to Los Angeles, San Diego or San Jose, each which sees over six thousand children per year and have two hundred social workers. Their budgets for child abuse and child neglect number around $350 million a year. Lake County $1 million because it is a retirement community and there's no money. Thus Lake County only opens cases involving severe molest, all incest, and all others have parental rights terminated for all perpetrating parents even if they do not reside in Lake County.

05-10-07 I went to the home to visit mother without S. This evening S. is staying over at a school friend's home. Mother says this is one of S.'s two friends who regularly come over. I asked what progress she has made in her therapy. She said she continues to ask her psychotherapist how long therapy is going to take. Her psychotherapist said they have to deal adequately with the protection issues. Her psychotherapist will not allow dad back in the home because S.'s therapist says he has severed the essential empathic bond. She feels she is being punished and Fred isn't. She says she took S.'s side immediately. The problem didn't occur by her husband.

I said that the attitudes governing the adults' relationships are at question. Because of what happened to her she should have assumed Fred could not be alone with S. nor spend an overnight at her house. That one relationship had to be protected against. Even after the night it occurred she should have disallowed any contact for extended family until it was first approved after I made a series of visits for a home study. She stated she felt she had that right because her case plan under the orders says, "visits to be arranged." I said that pertained to my authority once I ran a clearance. I said we discussed this with her lawyer present. She said she was granted custody; I said not yet, that S. is placed with her. She was unaware of that.

That afternoon I contacted each participating therapist. Their information was as follows,

05-10-07 Mother's therapist: sees client weekly for half hour, mother is making good progress but resents having to come. She has good ideas as to what her child requires. She has opened up a bit. She told her husband to leave, felt he would not protect. He is concerned that although angry at perpetrator family is financially dependent on him. Husband is dyslexic, can't find jobs easily. Has asked to meet husband, client not ready. He feels client has begun some parental alienation of S. wanting S. to view her mother as victimized. He will charge client for other half hour as soon as initial ten sessions are reached and then submit a brief evaluation, probably two paragraphs.

05-10-07 Husband's therapist says good patient, highly motivated. Pt. moved out of home upon wife's request after he said he thought she overreacted. He has moved in with Jim, goes to work with Fred. Jim introduced husband to wife. Husband sees wife's mother weekly for Wednesday breakfast at local cafe. Is financially paying for all costs related to S. Asked to cover wife's therapy. Problem here is husband said he wants to really screw Fred for what he did. He has sent husband for evaluation to assess him motivationally.

05-10-07 Child's therapist feels S. is overly parentified, she copes by confrontation. She says her mother does this. She says she feels safe. However she has had to come to understand her dad as someone who won't stand up to Fred. This has made her have a loss of confidence. While she doesn't say she hates him, she doesn't want to see him. He read his notes: "I don't care if he ever comes home, mommy is not in love, mommy says never get in Fred's car even if Jim is driving and Fred isn't in the car. Daddy wants me to like him but he doesn't do likeable things when he says he wants to marry Fred." This last part is the mother talking, not S.

05-10-07 Fred's therapist says Fred is there because otherwise judge will put him in jail. Fred is resistant. He says he did it to the mother and she came out alright, this was at age 16 for her. Fred doesn't seem able to acknowledge child is 11. Fred says his father raised him watching him have sex with dates. Fred was 12. He believes Fred is child's mother's first relationship and doesn't understand what he is still doing in her life. Tx does not think Fred will ever be capable of an apology session.

05-19-07 I met with S., her mom and her grandmother at the agency clinic for our scheduled session. I asked mom to tell S. about anything she is talking to her tx. Mom said she is working through a tendency to have people take her side instead of dad's. She doesn't like what happened and wished she had done a better job to make sure S. hadn't had to go through it. S. got teary. I asked grandmother to say how dad is, if she knows. She told S. she has lunch with dad regularly and he seems fine. Grandmother told S. she is rather annoyed at situation with dad because he wants to move in with her, to which S. said, then she could live there, and her mother turned to grandmother and said, "the least you could do is offer me a little support." I asked S. if she knows what they are talking about. S. said mom wants to return to school at night and grandma wants her to cut her hours and go mornings. Neither wants dad to know. I asked the two females about this. Grandmother said mom as good as she is won't let go of the past, mom wants controlling interests in Fred's company because she put it together.

Case B

The narcissistic patient usually presents as interesting, adept at scientific skills, in a turmoil intrapsychically, often unable to bring themselves to act on a reasonable plan that will keep them safe from harm. The following is excerpted from notes. The young male learned after the case was adjudicated that he had been named as the alleged father of my client's nine year old child. However she had not seen him in approximately a year.

"I am not altogether certain why I should be here except that I was referred for general counseling," the young male said, after a long pause for reflection. "I am a student at the university in my third year."
"What is your major?" I asked.
"Originally I intended to become a physician, but last year I changed my major to nursing. I think I'll do better. I can work an emergency ward when I'm done or go overseas. It's the job flexibility I really liked."
"What about becoming a physician decided you against completing?"
"My mother wanted me to become a nurse to begin with like her, but my dad's a physician. I thought I would do that, to be like him. I thought eventually I'd work with him in private practice, and then something happened. It's actually why I decided to come in."
"How did you choose to attend this campus? Were you raised here?"
"No, my mother moved to the area when I was about 18. Neither Laney nor Cal State had a school of internal medicine, so I applied here. I talked to an admissions counselor who tested me and thought medicine would be my best bet."
"Well, you would be in good company. Graduates from this campus do very well after they leave."
"Yes, I know, I was told that. The fact is I enjoy my studies although I'm not sure how I will put myself through school. I've

exhausted my finances."

"That must pose a hardship. Do you have a job?"

"I had a job but my mother insisted I give it up to focus more on my studies. I contacted my dad but he's retired and won't be able to send me more money."

"Do you have shelter?"

"Yes, we live in an apartment with her boyfriend. The problem for me is it is very small, about four hundred and fifty square feet, and my room is actually a large closet with a window. I didn't ever stop to think I wouldn't fit in."

"Tell me about your living situation."

"Well, we reside with him. He's lived here about ten years according to him, he attends the college also, he and my mother really hit it off. He's another nurse. He works for the Visiting Nurses and he said he could get me a job."

"That's definitely worth pursuing. Have you lived at home most of your life?"

"Yes, I'm very close to my mother. I have all her textbooks, her papers, and her tests," he said with a wry smile. "I really do study."

"I'm sure you do. So you grew up out here?"

"No, we're from the midwest. We had a ranch out there. I grew up there."

"What city would that have been?"

"Des Moines, Iowa."

"Friendly place. Lots of fields."

He seemed an affable male, knowledgable and aware. In addition, at the time, I didn't have many professionals studying at the University. He wanted to stay close to the campus and I decided he had other ties of some sort.

I said, "Have you ever seen a counselor before?"

"Only an academic one. He felt I ought to go parttime until I had a job on campus."

"I'd like to explain. I will see you once a week on any day of your choosing for fifty-five minutes. I ask that you talk about whatever you feel would be beneficial. My task is to facilitate awareness for you. We will evaluate after about ten weeks. If counseling is useful for you, we will continue. What day is good for you?"

"Mondays because I have just one class in the morning. I can come between one and five."

"Fine. I will meet with you here at four."

The next session was less awkward. He brought a copy of a court report he had received in the mail. He was not certain what his obligations might become.

I read the court report. "This is standard language. It says you were named by the mother as the male she slept with when she became pregnant. You can appear in court to request an order to be tested for paternity. Otherwise if you want to meet your child I can arrange that but you would then have to complete your plan first.

"Your case plan says you have only to be in counseling. You can do that here for awhile. When I believe you are ready to discuss parenting and custodial support, I will refer you. For that therapy you must pay fifty dollars an hour and be seen for a minimum of thirty sessions. Then that psychotherapist will submit their report to the court."

"That's alright with me. It's rather sudden. I knew this female for about a year during which time I had relations with her approximately three times a week. I felt she was too possessive. She wanted marriage. I said to myself that I was too young, I was 22. I just couldn't see supporting her and working my way through college."

"Lots of young males these days choose that. It's a large responsibility to take on. I think you've made some good decisions in postponing a decision like that. Going too fast can become a problem later."

"That's how I felt. I just wasn't ready. I spent lots of time thinking about kids and her and then told myself if anything happens to my mother or father, where would that leave me?"

"Those are very good thinking. How do you normally come about these decisions on any subject?"

"Well, I start with how I feel. If I don't get nervous then it's alright, but usually I try not to be the one to decide things. I ask my mother what she would do. I ask my friends at school. I ask my guidance counselor. Then I leave it alone for a long time."

"What causes you to want to become a parent now?"

"I thought I should consider if I should be supporting my child. I don't think it's right to not raise a child if one has one. I've always felt this way. I can't think what a child would think if he knew he had a father in the world who hadn't gotten to know him."

The task over time was to determine if he would be consistent with his stated intentions. This could be a guide to his abilities to sustain parenting through confusion, child rearing, parenting items.

"What do you think a parent should be?"

"I don't know. I guess I would have meals ready, drive him to and from school, take him on my chores, take him to school."

"Is there daycare at school?"

"No. I would have the receptionist watch him."

"You'd have to arrange babysitting. It's expensive. See if you can find a slot for almost no or little cost. Be certain you have the child when you are not in class."

"I just don't think I'd have much to contribute. I spend alot of time trying to figure out how I got started at this place. I just wind up thinking I should have stayed in Iowa. I think I had a nice life there but I'm a follower. I let my father lead me around by the nose."

"What sort of male was your father?"

"He was a military male stationed in Alabama for ten years. He was strict. He used to wake me at seven every day including weekends, make me shine my boots, clean my room, fold my blankets, eat breakfast, wash down the car, before I walked to school. He was stern, almost never any fun, insulted my friends, drove too fast."

"That seems to be a soft commitment. "

"That's the reason I follow my mother."

"How much older is your mother than you?"

He was taken aback. "Seventeen years."

"What makes you still live at home?"

"I have nowhere else to be."

"Why not move in with the child's mother and get to know the child?"

"I can't support her on my income."

"Why don't you let her support you temporarily?"

"I don't allow that. I am my own male."

"Does residing at home ever become intolerable?"

"All the time. It's why I am here. I need your opinion."

"I don't give opinions. I facilitate your decision making. The opinions are up to you."

He seemed to be playing at a game, satisfying someone else's requirements, not his preferred visa.

"I cannot tell if you are sincere or if you have a need to be told how to run your life, I don't have any interests in making your mind decide what will be for you."

"I was told, never make up your mind."

It seemed very unusual that a male of his age and professional study would relentlessly pursue a decision if he did not intend to ever decide to move forward. It was a preoccupation of the rich to stay put. He lacked means.

When I next met him he had shaved his head, wore a turban, was in boots and seemed a bit indecisive. He lacked the aura of energy he manifested. He was sullen, perhaps apprehensive, no longer what the nose would know. If he tracked others with an idea of how he might gain he would not be tracking in his garb.

"How is it you decided to change your clothing?"

"I thought over my last session, so I came today as I dress around the house."

"How does your mother and her man friend dress?"

"Always the same. He is in shorts, she wears a halter and a pair of pants. She likes him to stare at her. Why she does this I couldn't explain, I think she doesn't want me to think like a man."

"How do males think?"

"With their pants. Anything I do that starts here lands here."
"Do you mean that metaphorically?"
"Yes, I do. I wouldn't put myself in that position for any reason. I guess I didn't think to wear a condom. She said she was on birth control, I'm pretty sure. I assumed women take care of that sort of thing. After all, they have the pregnancy."

This medical student is age appropriate for the American culture at his age. The central issue here is not the material he is presenting although that material bears some indepth evaluation at a later time. My estimation for a second session is he requires plenty of psychological space to determine his own issues.

A third session produced a more focussed presentation. My client was a bit more forthright, but still not fluid in his responses, testing out what his actual position might be. It would become my task to discern if my client could look at his decision-making abilities.

"I made a decision. I'm going to complete my doctorate."
"What took you to that decision?"
"Well, I talked it over with my mother. She feels since I'm already in the program I should stay in through my internship. We discussed what I will do in ten years."
"Was this the first time you asked her opinion on this?"
"Yes, it was. Her boyfriend gave me that idea. He thought that since I was having so much difficulty I ought to enter nursing which might be easier. I considered it even though a job might not pay as much."
"What was difficult in medical school?"
"It was the amount of reading, the fact that I wouldn't be able to start my internship until I have completed my educational component, or I would have to take additional coursework later if I took a job as a nurse."
"Why would that be a problem?"
"Because," he said rather upset, "I have to demonstrate to the curriculum program that I understand the principles first. I feel I have a good grasp."

"Do you have a medical degree from a foreign government?"
"I have training from New South Wales."
"You could ask for your transcripts to be sent."
"The university has them."
"Then they must have counseled you."
"They did. I didn't think it could take long."
"Medical school goes for ten years in this country after which there is an internship of at least two years. It's a very long program."
"I just wasn't paying attention. It got away from me."
"Are you able to put any words to that feeling?"
He sat silently for a good minute. Finally, with heaviness, he said, "I think I counted on something happening that I shouldn't have."
I sat quietly also. Were I to have his experience, whatever it was, I imagined I would be disappointed in myself for failing to act or for having acted. Inward anger, deciding to do something he shouldn't, helplessness now, depressed.
Finally he said, "My mother who is only seventeen years older than me refuses to have me move out. She can't stand up to her boyfriend whom we live with. He likes to do things that I don't actually think are a good idea and I don't want to go far away from my mother."
"What does the boyfriend do that has you worried?"
"He dresses."
"As a female?"
"Yes. It bothers me."
"Similar to how you came to the last session?"
"No, he puts on makeup, a dress and heels."
"I can see how that could make you feel uncomfortable."
"Yes, it does, and he goes out in public that way. People who meet him don't realize they already know him."
"What do you think about that?"
"I think he should be honest with people he is friends with. I think he's trying to pull the wool over their eyes. When they come over, he tells them mean jokes making fun of what they've said. I can tell it embarrasses them. They try to remember to

whom they said that, they flash on something, then he gets mean. It's like he's always drunk."

"Does he drink alot?"

"Yes, so does my mother. They consume four bottles a night between them. Then they play loud music all night and wind up asleep on the floor. I feel I'm not wanted there. Half the time I find my mother so drunk I can't wake her."

"I agree that there is a serious problem. Have you considered your options?"

"No, I haven't. I guess I'd rather see my mother move out."

"Could she afford it?"

"I don't think she has any money since my father ran out on us."

"I've been rethinking my decision to continue with medical school. I've applied to nursing school and asked for my transcripts to be forwarded. The one thing I noticed is they have no electives in subjects I was taking. That would be geography, physical science, and elective math. Nursing would take a little under a year with no non medical coursework. I am told they will place me in a high paying job before I graduate."

"That was an excellent decision. I think you will eliminate a good deal of your worries when you start work. How do you find yourself feeling?"

"I expected to feel relieved, that I have a secure future. They gave me a tour of Pill Hill and after I thought, not anything I would do."

"I gather you wanted to work in a different setting."

"I had thought I could get a job on campus."

"I'm not aware of requirements for the teaching hospital. Had an advisor told you?"

"No, I know someone there. He suggested it."

"Does he hire?"

"Not anymore. That's the reason I got worried."

"That would worry anyone."

His eyes watered. He became self conscious, pulled at the sleeves of his scandanavian black and white sweater, crossed his legs. His trimmed crewcut and clean appearance looked for once vulnerable.

"I imagine it's disappointing to decide another course of intent is better after you've become so involved."

"That's not it." He sat for a long time stifling an emotion. "I wanted to give my mother her freedom and she doesn't want it."

"I think we ought to talk about this."

"I don't have alot to talk about. She's my mom. People used to kid us because she had me out of wedlock. She was young. When I was four my father left us. I know I should be on my own by now but I can't leave her. She gets real drunk and someone has to be there. Her boyfriend won't stay at home when she gets like this. He then goes out in drag and gets laid."

"How does your mother take it?"

"She flies into a rage. She accuses him of infidelity, she says he spends too much time out of the house, she calls him names and she slaps him and pulls his hair."

"That must take alot of psychic energy to know it's there. When this has happened have you been the person to calm her down?"

"Yes. There's no one else."

"How many years has this been her way of relating to you?"

"Since I was about eight or nine. I used to get a blanket for her after she fell asleep on the couch waiting for him to come home."

Perhaps he had learned something about someone he knew and did not know what he should do. This would be a straightforward case because the dynamic remains consistent and he is willing to look at it. His normative measures are a structure she relies upon to help stabilize herself. He still has to decide if he is willing to rear his son. At this stage of therapy the task is to have him sort through how he arrives at decisions. The process of talking about the thinking he attributes to his decisions is essential as a first step before he explores his emotions about his life experiences.

"You have given this issue alot of thought. Does it make you feel you are equipped to raise a child?"

"I don't know. I'm not sure I'd make a very good role model. I think I'm a nice person, I think I have good ideas. I like children but I don't permit myself to get angry. I don't feel comfortable around anyone who gets angry."

"Perhaps you want to ask for separate custody."

"Oh, I didn't know I could do that."

"Yes, you can."

"Can you recommend it?"

"Eventually."

"I don't think I would walk out on a child the way my father walked out on my mom. I would want my son always with me."

"That's a lifelong obligation. I commend you."

He smiled for the first time. "Thanks. I've never been told that by anyone."

"Not by your mother?"

"No. She wouldn't say that to me. I might say that to her if I felt she needed it."

"So in your friendship with your mother you're often her parent."

"No. She is my mother. I am her son. I was her child and she raised me. I don't make any false pretenses."

"At what age were you when she became drunk all the time?"

"Around 15."

"I see that all the time when children reach the age their parents were when they had them. Fifteen should have been for proms, a car, your first few dates, and so on."

"I've had just one girlfriend. She didn't like my mother."

"Is this the mother of your child?"

"No. Jane was a few months of love."

"What about your girlfriend?"

"I knew her for five years when we first moved."

"Around age 17?"

"Yes. She was my first. I stayed at her cabin with her in the country."

"Could you tell me about that?"

"Sure. She was very pretty. She had long blondish hair to her waist, she was a graduate of a two year minister program, her father ran a halfway house for alcoholics, she loved me completely."

"Why only five years?"

"My mother moved in with her boyfriend and asked me to come stay."

"Did you want to leave the cabin?"

"No. I wanted to stay forever. I once told myself if my mother were to be in trouble I would go to her without any questions asked."

"Did you see your friend again?"

"No. I became friends with Jane a year later."

"What are you feeling right now?"

"Tense, a bit apprehensive, unsure where you're going with this. I think I'm alright but I am aware I'm waiting for the other shoe to drop."

"Do you feel criticized by me?"

"No, I never feel that way with you. That's just what I am feeling."

"Alright. I asked because when I want to understand the feelings you experience with the remembrances you are having, sometimes people perceive of the realization as sudden and feel unprepared for what they feel."

"I don't know what I feel about most things."

"Being apprehensive might feel threatening if you aren't sure what the feeling is telling you about the situation."

At this point after the young man has connected an idea, his attitude about it, and attached a feeling, he is ready to begin this often emotionaally trying task once he has conscious practice at clarifying his thinking process. For this session during which he has empowered himself, he now has an instrument with which to examine his reactions and test his beliefs about them. The central issue as to his relationship with his mother is not the task of early sessions although it constitutes the subject matter. For this client to delve into this complex relationship he requires skills he has not yet developed. He does not yet see into the method of question and answer to define the information he wishes to glean.

A much later session, more revealing in content, delineates the parent/child dynamic despite the reality that the young man has wrestled with numerous emotional definitions as to tasks his mother enacts, his reactions and responses, and what tasks he endeavors with which to humor her. This session occurs a year into therapy. He has attended weekly missing not a session. He is prompt, works hard to think over what he is exploring for himself.

"My mother is pretty. She is blond, has wavy hair, it is layered with a bit of greyish brown, a little taller than myself, thin, thin through the arms and legs, sculpted cheekbones. She likes to sit at the window inside the breakfast nook, sip coffee and watch the neighbors get in their cars and go to work. She is usually chatty, likes to tease."
"What sort of things does she tease about?"
"She tousels my hair when it's wet and calls me her big boy."
"So you and she are the same height now."
"Yes," he was surprised, "we have been since I turned 17."
"This is when you went to live with your first friend?"
"Yes. My father left her a house and she sold it. She moved into a tiny condominium."
"Did you feel kicked out, because 17 is young to leave home?"
"Never thought of it that way. His house was huge but she couldn't keep it up, and that's her right."
"And you were in love."
"No. That was just fun."
"Is that upon retrospect?"
"Yes. At the time I thought Diane walked on water. She was a wonderful woman. She did everything and she loved me."
"Is it difficult to have known a person who loved you?"
He became saddened. "I didn't feel she needed me. She was just there. If anything I was dependent upon her."
"Was that financial or emotional?"
"Emotional. I could talk about things and she always knew what I meant. She aaccepted me for who I was. I didn't ask for much, I would have been happy to have a child with her but she used birth control." He paused; then said, "It's a place I get stuck in about Jane. She told me she was on the pill. She couldn't possibly have been."

"You sound to me a bit angry."

"No, I'm not. I wouldn't want my child to think I resented him."

"Do you think you're roped in for your future income?"

"Yes. I don't think I like getting stuck with the bill. Why hasn't Jane gotten herself a boyfriend yet?"

"Maybe the idea she has a child to support scares them off."

"She could go to Parents Without Partners. Lots of fathers roaming loose."

"It is a good social circle for single parents looking to take the cuff off loneliness and isolation."

"I guess I am angry. I despise women who do that."

"Have you known many?"

"No, not a one. I like women who don't want anything. They are just there. I can come and go without having to get bankrolled."

"There are men who say they want to be taken by their partner's pregnancies. For them that is an awareness they have possessed."

"I think I would leave a female for that."

I felt his intensity of newly realized anger had to be mirrored to him. After all this was his life. As a social worker I would not alienate him from his emotional status. I knew my boundaries. This was a complaint many social workers better than I wrestled with.

I said, "That's a strong indictment."

After a long silence, he replied, "That's why I don't choose to express anger."

I let a few seconds go by not to rush his process so he had lots of psychic space which I perceived rightly or wrongly he needed in order for him to become familiar with his adaptive behavior. "Anger is a good friend if you can learn to handle the coercive potential that you don't like about it."

"Anger wouldn't be my friend. Not after what I've seen."

"What have you seen?"

"My mother getting awakened in the middle of the night when John comes in. She gets up, corners him about where he's been, he lies and then she hits him. He grabs her wrists, tries to hold her off, and she kicks him."

"What did John tell her?"

"That he had been out all night at a gay bar."

"Did he ever indicate with you why he didn't go to a straight bar?"

"That's the only bar in the area. Otherwise he'd have to drive to the plaza. He walked down three blocks. He said he'd talk to guys at the bar, figure out how they tried to hit on a female and later try it on her. She loved it."

"Did you ever go with him?"

"No, I went with her. It's a nice clean nightclub, has a dance floor, a long very fashionable bar with mirror backed walls, a few billiard tables, serves expressos during the day, puts tables out on the sidewalk."

"What decided you to take her?"

"I thought if she saw where he spent his time, she wouldn't get so upset. But the problem wasn't ever that. I followed him."

Here we had a conflict of boundaries. He should not have taken this course of action on behalf of his mother's mistrust. There was possibly nothing she could do if John was actually having an affair as she feared, but if he were hooking or picking up a one night stand at a gay bar, she would need to know for health reasons if he was a carrier of HIV.

"Do you think that was wise?"

"Well, here's the deal. Maybe he should use a condom."

"I absolutely agree."

"I suggested it to him. He practically tore my head off. He said, I don't want you in my business, you just live here. This is my house. If I wanted I could put your mother on the avenue.

"I went to the bar he said he went to but he wasn't there. I then went to other bars. He wasn't there either. I made rounds of all the bars in the city. I was baffled. Finally I left the house when he did. I followed him on foot. He went to a restaurant that after nine becomes a nightclub. I took a table and watched for who would show up. A man showed up. I got up after I saw this act a few times, walked past their table."

"What is the job you got?"
"Oh, it's great. I work in a small group practice headed by a physician psychiatrist. I take vitals, I take a thorough medical history, draw blood, fill prescriptions and triage all day long. My supervisor is another nurse who has me doing chart review once a week. I don't actually do any billing but have to sign off. I've been there almost a month and my pay tops at $28.90 an hour. If I prove myself I can sponge during surgery and then take $40.50 an hour. The drawback is if I sponge I am permitted no moonlighting and only up to thirty hours a week."
"I'm really proud of you. What does your mother think?"
For the first time he laughed, relaxed. "I can support her but she won't agree. I figure it's time I found my own pad in the neighborhood."
"Have you celebrated?"
"No, not yet."
"You must be relieved."
"I am. I feel great for the first time in years. I find though I don't trust my own perceptions."
I elect not to be drawn in by his self negation. His frequent use of the words "I don't" in my estimation go with having learned what he believes is a social skill. It could be his mother's often heard complaint to anyone.
He then said, as if catching himself, "It sounds false, I know. My perceptions took a tumble with that bar stuff."
"In some perhaps undefined way you got let go of your own life with that situation."
"I shouldn't have followed him, but I thought he was having an affair with a gay man. I wanted to be able to protect my mother."
"You might look at situations for where your needs end and your mother's begin. You and your mother are close in age. You and she are the same height. She no longer resides with your dad.

It's a divorced parent and her son, but there must be some rules in your lives which more clearly define your roles."

"We have lots of rules. I'm not allowed to enter their quarters. My room is on the other side of the living room. We eat breakfast and dinner together except when John works. On weekends I sleep in, they go to visit his mother once a month or they have hangovers."

"Let's look at your relationship, what are mother issues, what are yours. Your mother lives with a boyfriend. You are only temporarily living with them in his home. You ought not to have been put in charge of your mother's safety, that's for her to decide. Where do you think this confusion started?"

Another session at a year and three months gave the client his decision regarding his child who he brought with him. The child of four looked identical to him. Dressed in navy trousers and a pink shirt with collar and bolero and black boots, his light brown hair neatly parted and combed, he was every bit his father. They sat side by side, calm, attentive.

"What's your name?" I asked.
"James."
"How old are you?"
He held up four fingers. "Four."
"Has your father told you about me?"
He gave a nod.
"We have to talk about you and your dad. Your dad wants you to live with him at his house. Does he talk to your mom?"
"Yes, every day. He calls her and she talks to me."
"What does he talk about?"
"Our trip to the zoo. He gave me a zoo book."
"What is a zoo book?"
"It has a picture of every animal at the zoo. My mom reads it to me at night."
"Was that your idea?"
My client said it was. "I've arranged to take John two nights on the weekends. John's been to my home twice."
"Have you seen your dad's house?"

A nod. "I have my own room. Dad gave me lots of toys."
"What do you do at your dad's?"
"We go shopping, we eat dinner, we see TV, he gives me a bath."
"I've also taken him to a children's matinee, to the park, and I signed him up for daycare two hours on Saturday so he can play with children his age. I plan to invite another parent and child to join us at the park."
"Would you like that?"
The child answered in the affirmative.

I put in my evaluation a series of recommendations to the court. I suggested a plan of gradual increased visitation as to dad, to begin with weekend visitation after he gave the agency the name of the daycare group, that the agency pay for daycare if dad had to work, that all arrangements be made between the parents by telephone in advance of visits, and transfer of custody between parents may occur in person when the other parent picks up the child. I also recommended the client was to be seen biweekly in counseling with his son in order to assess for parent/child attachment.

Let's discuss the method for assessment, interview and evaluation with this population. Most professionals without training to assess clinically will not be able to help a client who has never been to a therapist learn to successfully utilize therapy. Because so much of child abuse occurs within a very complicated family dynamic it may not occur to the professional to meet with an entire family in order to assess if the parents or guardians have adequate control over their children and can supervise them. The issues that must be continually evaluated over time are parent/child attachment and empathy, the parent's ability to provide adequate supervision in the home of all children including teens, the parent's ability to create a meaningful structure of activities so the child as he or she grows up has a positive concept for family cohesion, a value system, morality, sex role mirroring, tangible goals and non corporal discipline. Also important are regular contact with a responsible supportive adult support network, problem solving, a plan for when something unanticipated comes along, and a contact person the child knows.

Psychological safety is the foremost consideration for governing adequate adult supervision of the child. This criteria is determined by several hallmark managed custodial items: that the child is not placed in a setting which reintroduces trauma, that the child is permitted the experience of a multitude of experiences under the watchful eye of a supportive adult, that the child is not exposed to either statements or inappropriate behaviors that would cause him or her to feel unsafe. Thus the parent should not leave the child unattended for long periods, ought not to say things that are prejudicial or create a chaotic environment that could produce harm or become harmful.

Emotional abuse differs from psychological safety because it involves a process of subjugation over a long period of time, often in excess of a year. This is difficult for the court to make a finding from allegations. Emotional abuse is usually believed to derive from negative remarks which over time cause a child to lose self esteem and to fear the primary caregiver. A parent who tells the child that he "is a no good loser who cannot do anything right" or who locks the child in a closet without food and water for over a day is guilty of such abuse. Generally if a petition citing emotional abuse cannot be sustained, a finding of neglect can be made.

The standard initial interviews must focus mostly on the adult's and conversely the child's perceptions of those situations that constitute the trauma. If there are a series of traumatic incidents, it must conform to what is known and alleged at least by the minor child. This process can be facilitated by the police or by a psychosocial evaluation performed by a school psychologist or a practicing psychologist or therapist. Once the trained social work professional has met and talked to the child, he or she must first ascertain why the parent thinks they are there.

Case C

"So what brings you into the system?"
"I was accused of trying to beat my youngest child."
"How old is he?"
"Tommy is seven."
"Can you tell me what the allegation says?"
"I'll show you the court papers." The twenty year old female pulled out a tiny folded paper, slowly opening it, and handed me the legal sized page.

I read it aloud. "'On or about January 10, 1998 the parent was observed to yell at the minor, slap him across the face causing redness, grab him by the hair and slam him against a car door in a parking lot at MacDonalds. When the parent was attempted to be restrained by two observing adults, the parent said, 'That's my bastard kid, leave him alone or I'll knock the shit out of you,' one adult called for the State police."

"Yes," the parent admitted, "I don't think they should have done that. Tommy is my kid."

"Had you ever struck Tommy before this time?"
"A few times. It's the way I was raised."
"Did you have custody of your son?"
"No, my ex does. I get him every other week on weekends."
"I gather the child was removed from your care. Were parental rights terminated?"
"No, I was told to enter counseling, meet with you, take two parenting classes."
"Do you have that order with you?"
"I left it at home."

This information you obtain for this initial interview must conform to the known findings made by the court. The information has to become a foundation from which you will help the client evaluate their behavior over time.

There should be a minimum of five interviews before any work can begin by you. Even if the parent or the parents have entered therapy, begun parenting class, or any other court mandate, you will still have to learn from the individual what their understanding is. Thus a first assessment might be formulated as the degree of compliance the client agrees to as demonstrated by his attitude, statements and how prepared he is. Each of your series of initial interviews should focus on the following tasks: obtain a basic understanding from the parent of his or her situation, set about to orient the parent as to what your participation is and rules for compliance, begin to establish raporte with the parent by having them describe their own upbringing, learn about when they married and why they chose the other parent, and what they think about their child. As to this last objective, you need to inquire what they believe a child who is their child's age is capable of, what type of guidance and instruction a child his age ought to have, who should provide it and what arrangements exist in case of emergencies. If the parent answers only with short quips, you might also discuss what the parent has begun to learn in parenting class. Ask to see their notebook and answers, find out who teaches the course, try to learn what other parents in the class are asking questions about. If your client appears belligerant, demanding or otherwise uncooperative, you can end your sessions and send a memo to the court. If your client has started to honestly look at any issue, you can solicit additional information by asking them to define their personal objectives for work with you. They should be willing to say they want their relationship with their child reinstated, how they think their behavior should be different and obstacles they feel contribute to previous incidents.

The interviewing questions should be open ended. This means that questions should not be able to be answered by one word. To learn to do this, write your questions out in advance.

What were you told about child rearing when you were in your teens or early twenties? Who had the biggest influence on you?

Please describe anyone in your family behave in irrational behaviors. What was your response?

Please describe people you know who are your friends. What are they like?

Do you feel you are in control of yourself when you are annoyed or impatient?

What happens when you lose your temper? If you drink or use drugs daily, what causes you to become less inhibited?

Do you sit on your anger letting it explode?

Do you think you are an abusive person?

A thorough history also should be obtained during an early interview about drug use, extramarital affairs if pertinent, incidences of domestic violence, mental health problems of a parent, work history and other problems.

Once these interviews have been conducted you must assess whether the client is willing to engage in therapy. Any unwillingness should be brought immediately to the court's attention. A request to terminate parental rights may be made. A new petition can only be submitted if the parent has injured the child under another section of the law.

It takes about eight months to establish a trusting interaction with a parent. During this time the parent should have become accepting of a therapeutic process with you and be willing to be seen weekly by their therapist by whom they have been seen. They will have a sufficient understanding of how counseling is to occur, the tasks they need to focus on, they will have gained understanding of normal age appropriate behavior for children, they may have had supervised visits with the child's therapist or a trained parent aide, and they will have returned to court for a six month review with a court report that discusses their progress on their case plan.

The next four to seven months will necessarily become family sessions in your monthly contacts when you visit. These monthly interviews should involve as many family members as possible. At this point you will have done each or all of the following:

- had face to face visits with the child
- obtained a medical on the child
- attended a school conference or an Individual Education Plan
- obtained a record of grades for the child with truancies
- talked to the therapist for the child
- talked to each therapist for each parent
- met with the custodial parent together with the child
- maintained the file

With a regular reporting system either from or to therapists and educators, a social work professional shall have an idea as to the parent's consistency and intention for constructive change. The clinical milestones at this juncture are:

- obvious insight into his own past behavior
- lessening of rigidly maintained ideas
- increased tolerance of ambivalence
- less coersive, belligerent or abusive manner
- an ability to identify with the child from a child's perception
- an understanding of parenting principles and knowledge of age appropriate behavior of children
- an understanding of a parent's age appropriate supervision of the child

In order for the court to grant a parent with reinstated parenting privileges the parent must change their behavior such that abuse is not likely to reoccur. This must be observed consistently by all parties who have contact with the parent. With partial compliance but no insight into his behavior nor newly adapted behavioral changes, the court will not give this parent any further contact with the minor.

For the parent who displays a willingness to change these four to seven months consist of necessary milestones:

- the parent must complete a letter in which he can tell the child he apologizes for past abusive behavior
- he must be able to receive questions the child has about his past behavior
- he must state how therapy has allowed him to change
- he has to be interviewed by the child's therapist and the primary caregiver's therapist
- he must have eliminated abusive language from his vocabulary
- he must have evolved a constructive method for handling his anxiety
- he must have undergone a treatment program if he was addicted to drugs or alcohol

If the treating therapists feel he has accomplished significant strides he is then asked to meet with the child and read his revised apology letter. The child is invited to ask him a question. He is then asked to leave. Several sessions are given to helping the minor think over the apology. If the child does not feel threatened, supervised visits by the child's therapist begin.

During this period the social work professional must again meet more often with the parent to assess him for ways he reports he is putting his changed behavior and insights into practice. He is advised to join a psychotherapy group in order to evaluate his new style of interaction. He must be able to display observable behaviors.

- tolerance for other people's ideas, disagreements and experiences
- refrain from dominating a group, be forthright, not attempt to be a bully or coersive, incorporate other people's successes, and think through his plans
- receive criticism and respond kindly
- accept a leader's guidance

In addition he should enter couple's therapy with the child's parent to arrange supportive plans for transportation to and from visits, daycare, babysitting, child complaints and other concerns which could include parents-in-laws, siblings, getting the child to school, setting up after school activities and sports or special interests.

In a case that is open to the court for a year, the social work clinician will conduct an average of 35 interviews each lasting one or more hours, up to four hours. The interviews that last several hours are conducted approximately every two or three weeks to stem crises for many situations.

- Teen incorrigibility or hostility toward a parent or guardian
- A family crisis
- A teen who has threatened a family member
- A hospitalization or 5150
- An acting out histrionic teen
- Coaching a parent in how to set limits for a child

Case D

If a family member must be seen weekly or several times a week the number of interviews within a three month frame may equal 35 times. Total interviews for these intensive cases averages several hundred hours from start to finish. Whichever reason your case has necessitated indepth weekly interviewing assessments, at around eight months a typical interview for physical abuse might be as follows:

"So you've exhausted your ideas."
"Yes. I draw a blank when I come here. I feel I am done with my work with you."
"We talked about a review last session. What did you do with that?"
"I gave it thought. I looked at my life, I've come a long way."
"Yes, you have. How was your group?"
"It went alright, I guess. I'm feeling bored. I've been through the stuff the rest are getting to there. I remember all the things I went through. The guy who runs it won't let me give advice so I tune it out."
"What's it like to just sit there and wait?"
"Nerve wracking. I can't stand the silences. They're wasted time."
"Do you think you'd feel better if the leader moves discussion along?"
"I guess you see this alot."
"I see all sorts of things. Advice giving, anger, controlling, people who leave. What do you tell yourself about someone else's process?"
"I don't know. I can't pull it out."
"Have you ever gone through this before?"
"I just don't want to have to wait on someone else to get there. I have my life."
"It's good to get it over and done with."
He cracked a grin. "No, I haven't ever been through it like

this. We waited over ten minutes for someone to say something."

"Must have been agonizing."

He gave another easier smile. "I don't know what I should think. I can't simply sit there and stare at them."

"What does your inner child say about it?"

"I told you, no inner child." He paused. "I begin to feel useless. I mean I spend alot of time by myself when my kid isn't with me or I watch TV. I can't figure it out, why it's a problem. It's like he has a fly on his nose."

"Many people think silence indicates a loss of interest."

"Or a nervous breakdown."

"How about we sit here without talking."

We sit in silence for five minutes.

I break the silence with, "How is that?"

"It's difficult. I don't know what you're thinking about me."

"Men who hit children reach a frustration peak more quickly than others. They find it almost impossible to contain their anxiety. They decrease this perception by altering focus and shifting attention to someone with less power over whom they think they have control and then blame them for an eventual loss of disciplined reserve."

The parent with the problem of physical abuse has already a poorly focussed discomfort with anxiety. He may have reached for the wine. He may have an overworked self blamer which tells him silence says something that can't be controlled with any predictable outcome. Although most people with normal behaviors have self critics and although the belief that people who commit domestic violence are raging men with grandiose borderline psychological conflicts, in this setting most people who will inflict emotional abuse on a young child suffer from an inability to release anxiety.

Case E

Public Services Officer: "Hello, my name is Judy Koretsky and I will be your services specialist for the next year. In my capacity I will arrange to meet with you and your family at a suitable time for approximately an hour during which I will review your progress on your plan and find out how things are going in the home. For starters I am interested to learn how you are this evening."

Mother: "We're fine, actually better than expected. Things have been financially very tight for months but Bob started working again."

Public Officer: "That must be a tremendous relief. Where do you work, Mr. Brown?"

Father: "I used to be an auditor for the county but my new job is as a general manager for materials management."

Public Officer: "Are the hours satisfactory?"

Father: "Oh, very, 8:00 am to 4:30 pm. I can drop Jean off at school and pick her up and take her with me to my AA meeting at the Fellowship on Thursdays."

Public Officer: "That sounds like a good use of time. How do you like your dad's AA group, Jean?"

Jean: (She is ten.) "I like it alot. Everyone's real friendly and they always say nice things to me. As soon as our church gets an Alanon group started, I'll be going to both."

Public Officer: "It seems you're doing alright this evening, Jean. How has she been getting along at school, Mrs. Brown?"

Mother: "We signed her up for an afterschool class for arts and crafts every day but Thursday so Bob and I can see the couple's counselor. It's working out well. Tell the lady about your field trip, honey."

Jean: "It was heckabad. We went on a bus to the museum. We pet the snakes, fed the bunnies and held the fish."

Public Officer: "Petting museums are great. Did they have a velvet felt room?"

Jean: "Yes. They had lots of neat patches, like zippers, velcro, purses, all sorts of neat things."

Mother: "I don't know if you know but I also work. I volunteer at Jean's school in the afternoons so I can see her and she can see me. Then I'm at my cashier job at the bowling alley from 2:30 pm until 9:30 pm at night. It takes me about twenty minutes to get home."

Father: "Mother has been looking for another job but the pay is alot where she works. She takes home about five thousand a month."

Public Officer: "That's an excellent wage. Have you been there long?"

Mother: "Eight years. I went back to work when Jean was old enough for daycare. Bob's mother had been living with us but she had to enter a nursing home a month ago."

Jean: "I miss her. She read me a bedtime story every night."

In this interview basic custodial care is readily evaluated. The child has a good relationship with her parents who interact spontaneously with her and with each other. Jean is well mannered, age appropriate with good observation. The problems areas are acknowledged. The father is the primary caretaker, he arranges transportation, is off work when the child is ready to be picked up, has dinner with her and spends evenings with her, getting her a nightly bath and putting her to bed. The mother has a schedule which prevents her from seeing to the child's needs most week nights.

In this family the petition was sustained for neglect. Substance use as to mother could not be proven for lack of evidence. Amphetamines only with a prescription are legal; otherwise they are considered illegal drug use. The mother's babysitter had her boyfriend over most evenings when Father worked. The boyfriend was aggressive and during arm wrestling fractured Jean's arm. As a result of the incident these parents are reluctant to hire in a young adult who will look after Jean responsibly. The absence of Bob's mother who probably oversaw the home is a major recent change that the family has not yet responded to.

Because these parents are considerate it is anticipated they will prove good candidates for treatment. Services are expected to be brief, with a new sitter or other arrangements in place soon. However a central question is mother's job and whether she uses drugs at all while she works. The referrant was an associate who is the daughter of Bob's mother's sister. Whereas she maintained that mother periodically seems tipsy late at night she was unwilling to furnish a statement for the court and three substance tests were negative.

In this curriculum it has to be understood that among the intern population as well as the licensed therapists who may provide therapy or parent or alcohol or abuse domestic violence education, this group may in fact seek employment with contracting service agencies, may provide education with a therapeutic component or may simply be working with families who require guidance in order to effectively simulate integration of counseling they are already receiving.

The method for inspiring insight begins with a matter-of-fact, easy back-and-forth raporte. While much of the evaluation is elicited through the appearance of normal conversation, the social worker must by the end of this initial interview understand the family dynamics and any threat to family stability. The parents on the other hand are required to demonstrate cognizant recognition that the incident that occurred remains in their control to fix. As they start a process for looking at when they might have known a problem existed prior to the petitioned situation they need to account for why they overlooked the information.

Public Officer (has just asked the child to leave the room) "I'm sure you're aware that the court would like you to be as involved as you can be in your participation. The bureau hopes to have you come up with a plan of communication with Jean which you feel can help you assess whatever you need so as to keep or change a plan for daycare. Thus the work ahead lies with a mutual effort to identify what you feel Jean can say because she is just a young child."

Mother: "It shouldn't involve much. Jean stays up Friday

nights to hear about my evening. She's usually forthcoming."

Father: "When mother got off at 7:30 pm Jean and I used to drive there to pick her up."

Public Officer: "How was it for Jean to see your office?"

Mother: "I was often on the lanes by then. A friend of mine was injured and I added on part of his time onto my check."

Father: "Jean thinks of her mother like a shining star. She is a pro, sells balls, works the tournaments. Once a season she enters on a team."

Mother: "This won't be the first time I've asked myself if she should stay up that late or if she should see me when I can't really stop and chat with her. There's a great deal of clubbing around. I'm just not sure how much is good for her to be exposed to."

Public Officer: "What activities don't you want her to see?"

Father: "She has a good time. She sips soda, plays a round, gets rather chummy. When she's at the register she's all business, she's busy, harried in fact, gets snappish. She doesn't talk. Jean mistakes that behavior for moodiness."

Mother: "Jean was down once when I had to bartend. The usual couldn't come."

Father: "That was the weekend we asked the babysitter to pick her up. It was getting pretty wild. We can't seem to find reliable help."

Public Officer: (Meets with Jean's parents at the clinic) "These test results found a low amount of amphetamine in your system. Is this a recent use?"

Mother: "This man at work drops by once a month. He gives each of us working girls a tab. I use it infrequently, it's not enough to get hooked. We have an employee birthday for these occasions and after we have a few drinks and then a meal. I'm surprised it even showed. How much was it?"

Public Officer: "90 mg. We didn't find for alcohol."

Mother: "I'd be happy to test for you. I really wouldn't want anyone to think I have a problem. I'm the one who invited my mother-in-law down when we were having problems. We used to drink at the bar at the alley Saturday nights until the sitter came in with Jean after a movie. The alley had finished a tournament, everyone was loaded. I looked at myself in the mirror, thought I was haggard and over the hill and then Jean caught my gaze. I just didn't react for a moment until I saw her steady hand Jean a drink. I went and got Bob. I had a flash that Jean could be me, married at 19, a child at 20, almost no skills, having to take a local job, never making it out of this pit."

Father: "I didn't know you used, Mother. Has Jean ever seen you at it?"

Mother: "I had just slipped myself a half tab that night while I was waitressing. That was immediately before I went to check my face."

Father: "When we got home the sitter was watching TV and her boyfriend was bandaging Jean's arm after having done some arm wrestling. I took Jean to the emergency."

Public Officer: "I would like to arrange some random tests for you over the next month. While 90 mg is not alot, it has the potential to become very addictive."

Mother: "That's probably a good idea. I don't use as a rule except when we have birthdays at work. I don't think of myself as that type, but I do want to be sensitive to the concern. If it weren't for the people I work for, it wouldn't be there at all. I guess the item is I'm the youngest staff there and without the job we're dead. Bob's pay by itself won't take care of the bills. I don't feel the freedom to say no. None of them are users or whacked out, I don't expect that to occur with me. I hear you, though, I can't afford to make it a thrill."

This is a common situation in denial of alcohol or drug use. Because the use is minimized, the problem appears trivial. In order for the referral by the aunt to be evaluated as to actual risk to the child, amount and frequency of use has to be discussed for every occasion used. The problem becomes identified when the parent, in this case the mother, can match the descriptions given by the referrant and the husband. When this mother can say to the boss' friend that she is in recovery and cannot partake of the drug, she will have figured out how not to jeopardize her clear thinking and judgement, both which control her interactions to her child.

Many insights are small. A few will be major insights. These will occur over time, rarely all at once. Since the function of gaining insight into what has shaped the client's attitudes and behaviors is to enable the client to become more sincere and flexible as an interactive rational thinking person, it stands to reason that when the client has an insight it will provide instantly a sense of humanistic relief. The benefit of insight then may be said to provide progress to enhance their journey in the discovery of Self. It is the discovery of one's nature and who one can become — better able to tolerate stress and confusion, more empathic oneself, more humanistic - that gives the person the ability to provide a contientious upbringing for their child.

Masterson, 1983, discusses the difficulties in treating borderline and narcissistic clients. He describes a continual testing of the therapist's authority with regard to scheduling office appointments, taping sessions, transference and countertransference, social standards of dress, fee for treatment and a host of other complaints from clients for whom the essential parent/child attachment was disrupted at an early age. Mahler, 1985, offers a working definition for the normative development for ages six months to three years to explain necessary psychological functions for parent/child attachment and bonding. At an early age the newborn is held, fed, cuddled and spoken to. These parenting tasks are accompanied by constant eye contact, expressions of love and being held. At one years when the baby learns to crawl and sit, the parent is in careful attendance providing support and tenderness. At age two when it would be appropriate for a child to be placed in a crib for brief periods, in those relationships in which there has been ambivalence about being a parent, the disruption of attachment is thought to begin. Horner cites that the parent who leaves and who does not come back emotionally is thought to produce a borderline and that the parent who is absent emotionally until they come back after brief periods produces a narcissist. Horner states that these messages become internalized within the psychological mapping of the toddler as this primary relationship between parent and child continues.

There is much controversy as to whether either presentation is capable of any real change once this imprinting has occurred. Some therapists evaluate the client by any ability to change. The individuals who can are said to have a trait; those who remain fixed in this disrupted attachment syndrome are believed to be unable to change and can only be managed. These clients require a good deal of structure. Therapy usually lasts about three years, possibly longer if they will commit. Some require being seen twice a week. The goal of therapy is to form a rigid structure such that essential concerns are always addressed in the same way, permitting the client to eventually adapt by introjecting aspects of the structure of the relationship. Thus, it is expected that for a client whose defense of their personal ego identity is dominated by continual rage, the introject of any part of the therapeutic structure - showing to appointments on time, sitting five feet away from another person, paying a portion of household costs, selecting one's choice of clothing, making a few decisions oneself - will give the client a sense of self mastery and confidence, allowing the defense to become less engaged. Over a year of weekly sessions the client may become less dependent and more self fulfilling.

For a narcissistic client who belies a need to be seen as very attractive or seductive, the defense of the self is to ward off anxiety by drawing people toward a pseudo self. Thus the narcissism comes across as an individual who was not loved enough, unlike the borderline who although they may have been loved there is an all pervasive sense of emptiness or lack of personal significance. A narcissist is not likely to rail against structure as much as against the appearance of an inability to draw the therapist into the idea of a complication to the essential relationship. For this person the test of his or her capable self mastery may be to enable the therapist to view him as special, whether the therapist does this is not made part of realism. Complexities for this client may consist of queries such as, how well does the therapist view him, is the therapist able to transcend as the client would like, can the therapist be trusted, etc.

Within the realm of family dynamics there are likely to be a large number of these clients. Borderlines tend to create instability for their children, narcissists tend to use drugs or alcohol to increase their social flair. If the parent has an essential psychological injury the child is likely to be taught the same lack of ego identity as was learned by the parent.

The ability to have honest insight becomes complicated when the parent lacks a real sense of identity. In order for the parent to be somewhat free of hankering doubts, a good place to start therapeutically is in a therapy education group. The focus soon falls away from the individual and begins to become squarely placed on the dynamics of the group or class. Emptiness is replaced by concern; not having enough attention is replaced by the normative questions every member asks themselves. After a six month group there has been sufficient emotional risks taken such that these clients can be seen for individual work and be able to risk additional personal disclosure.

If the parent is unable to find a therapy group nearby, the grouping can consist of the family with whom the child lives and extended family members, depending upon their availability. In addition in order to test degree or dimension of insight the therapist can arrange the following combinations yearly:

- all adults for each family of the case plan for discussions as to supervised or extended visitation, trips, and overnights;
- all adults involved with the court case, attorneys and treating therapists for changes in the law that might affect the child's placement;
- all treating therapists and children for the family of the case plan to discuss progress and therapeutic goals; and
- the child or children for whom school conduct is reviewed, all teachers, tutors, and treating therapist.

Toward the end of the case plan implementation these sessions can be used to sign off on agreements. These agreements can then become a final outcome report submitted to the court to attest to the judge that the petitioned facts are resolved.

The Process of Gaining Insight

The initial start of rehabilitation in a public service case is the naming of the facts. An event consisting of risk of harm to a minor occurs. A referral is made to the social work desk. The central coordinator rates the risk as either an immediate or a ten day and then assigns the referral for investigation. For an immediate risk the investigator has twenty-four hours to complete the investigation; if the risk is past or deemed less than severe the investigation must be completed in ten days. All investigations yield evidence consisting of but not limited to a police, sheriff, or a physician report stating an injury was observed on the minor, interviews with witnesses having knowledge of the incident, and/or previous orders, psychosocial assessments and other pertinent information. If cause is found to be sufficient, a petition stating the allegations is filed within the same time frame. Once the hearing is commenced the judge then sets a date for juris to hear and find true part or all of the allegations or sets the matter for trial if the person against whom the petition is filed argues or denies. Before this process of identifying the problem can be rehabilitated there must be findings to substantiate the facts are true and that the minor falls under a legal definition as to age and cause.

Rehabilitation is determined by the case plan. This plan says what must be completed in order for the parent or guardian to resume custody of the minor. During this period the minor may reside in someone else's care. For each type of allegation certain services must be entered into and either on the way to being completed or completed before the court will make a new order. The most frequent petitions are sustained for physical abuse resulting in marks, welts or injury; neglect during which the child was harmed or at risk of harm because the parent was absent or neglectful; emotional abuse causing the child to decompensate or otherwise seriously regress; sex abuse; and abandonment in which the parent left the child and did not return for him or her. The plan will state that the parent must enter into therapy, attend a parent education group of at least 8 hours, enter into group or family therapy after successful completion of a parent education class and visit the child by arrangement designated by the social work professional.

The first interview must therefore answer the following consideration, when asked to state the reason the family is in the system is their answer consistent with the facts of the case? If the parent gives an explanation which provides the already stated facts of the case, it may be assumed that the rehabilitation can begin. However if the parent states they do not either agree with what occurred during the hearings, they must be referred back to their counsel. A subsequent meeting with parent and attorney is recommended in order to clarify what the parent's actual understanding is. At that meeting referrals to agencies outside the bureau should be given along with deadlines by which time each service must have begun. If they fail to comply a new petition citing refusal to comply is filed and if the minor is under age three an order for termination of parental rights and a request for adoption will be signed by the judge.

Once the parent agrees the sustained facts of the case are accurate, the interview should include a thorough review of at least one document. One is the disposition report containing the plan. This document should be read out loud to the parent and the information discussed as to the parent's comprehension of what is required.

As stated earlier the social work professional is expected to provide advisement on a regular basis to assure the court that the parent is making progress on their case plan. In order to provide this assurance the professional must conduct a minimum of one to two interviews each month with the child, each parent and the family together. During each interview the following information must be obtained: what is being discussed or looked at in their therapy, what information they are learning in their parenting class, results of testing if tests for sobriety are required. Additionally the child's immunization records should be noted for documentation in the file, there should be a recent medical examination and the child's attendance and grades also obtained. If the child has a tutor a verbal progress assessment can be made. For small children with any low apgar standard or medical difficulty, an assessment sould be done for a public health nurse to conduct inhome observation. There should also be an interview with the family to observe the dynamics of their interactions over time to assess emotional warmth and nurturing guidance, appropriate supervision, structure within the home, and special child activities.

Insight is a discovery of one's own response that provides one with clarification to usually their behavior or how someone else's behavior has affected them. In order to have insight, one has to have given thought to the critical factors that have molded one's responses. Thus, as a parent is trying to cope with the past experience of stress and betrayal, as he or she sifts through patterns of behavior and brings that emotional response close, the parent begins to appreciate or at least accept the overall act that has created detriment to the minor. The process of
acceptance may begin with understanding the fact of the petition: the husband who is the biological parent of a five year old son has slapped him leaving redness on his arms; as stepparent of a prepubescent teen, aged twelve, he has touched her

inappropriately in the mid-afternoon by touching her back and kissing her on the neck while dancing to the radio. The next part of the coping process involves saying how the act was perceived and the emotional damage done to the child. At this time, this mother is capable of an insight, such as, she has always prided herself on keeping a safe, trusting parent/child home but she has not been there to protect her children and the person whom she left in charge is abusive. She has left unquestioned her husband's frequent alcohol use. Remarks that indicate insight may be stated as follows: I gave over my power; our household is set up with Ron making all the decisions that affect each child; I shut out rational behavior when I become seized by vindictive anger and I go blank; I have to teach myself not to react that way. I like to regard myself as polite but I can no longer close myself off to the obvious – my live-in partner is too unhealthy and immature to be a reciprocal parent.

Thus, insight helps the previously unaware parent to regain lost ground. It facilitates freeing oneself from the harm that has been imposed upon the family. A child has a right to expect age-appropriate affection, and the parent has an obligation to assure that the child's rights of protection, guidance and safety are not invaded.

How The Client Has An Insight

The process for insight involves several mechanisms which as they become integrated by the client for early self acceptance signify a greater awareness and ability to self evaluate. These mechanisms are:

> (a) **reflective listening** - which begins as the therapist holds the client in high esteem by looking for strengths and ideals as defined for positive self regard by Carl Rodgers, a client in turn often responds with keen interest of promise of unlocking doors of problems,

> (b) **therapeutic modeling** - the therapist models behaviors such as sitting with silences, asking questions about

feeling states, learning what the client believes is of value from various classes, the therapist asks for feedback about therapy - how's it going, what do you hope to get out of it, how are you responding, a client might respond with impatience, it's taking too long, therapy wears me down, no one explains things,

(c) **empathy** - the therapist is empathic saying anger can be a helpful ally, what is your anger about?

(d) **transference, as defined by Jung** - the client has hope that they are not judged, feels accepted, begins to share experiences, the therapist comments on some material to offer containment, saying those experiences are universal, it's natural to feel that way, when people are raised around an abuser they shut down, try not to think, try to accomodate by repressing responses; the client puts to the therapist projected responses for which the feeling state may be rejected as something they elicit or feel;

(e) **therapeutic self adaptation** - when this occurs the therapist encourages the client to look at issues, how were they raised, what were they told about roles and rules and other people, what assumptions about the world were conveyed, who in the family insisted on being right, was client ever allowed to be in the right,

(f) **raporte** - after client has been easily unloading and commenting about things they are talking about, raporte is thought to be established, this is at about 6-8 months of therapy,

(g) **transparency as a goal of therapy** - the therapist can now begin introducing issues, insight can only happen with a person who wants to be honest with themselves; along with the client openly disclosing honest reactions, the therapist should be looking at: *what constitutes psychological safety for you; the therapist talks about this for as long as it takes for person to state what this is for themselves:

* do you find yourself giving into all or nothing thinking or idealizing people and subsequently devaluing them, that person is great, can do no wrong, the other one is a loser, this is a rejected part of themselves, a goal is to get them to define what undesirable aspect this could be, most likely it is some attribute the client doesn't want to associate with, being castigating, being overly dependent, feeling helpless,

* do you have an image of a nurturing caregiver, which parent is this, is this the same parent who abuses; with what type of person are you drawn to for female friendship, for male friendship, for sexual attraction, what qualities do you dislike in others, what qualities do you dislike in yourself.

(h) **psychological boundaries** - where do you begin and end, what information tells you this, when does this issue become unclear for you, when do you feel controlled by another individual, what do you think is going on, what responses are triggered.

These then constitute the process by which the client's behaviors are shaped as the material for each session is discussed. The client will by the tenth or eleventh month of therapy have had at least a half dozen insights. Some insights may be small, for example the client recognizing a mean parent had a certain impact long before domestic disputes erupted into violent acts.

Literature Review

The group systems modality is not meant for individuals with somatic disorders nor for those with fixated or entrenched pathologies including severe anxiety or threats to their well functioning. (Paul and Bernstein, 1973) Although there may be persons with degrees of anxiety response which pose maladaptive triggers to desired goals, whereas some victims and parents may present with various post-traumatic stress disorders, because many situations of child abuse naturally elicit an intrapsychic frozen anesthesia, the essential motivation for group work is to examine the obstacles to unlearning rigidified behaviors that have thwarted optimum functioning. (APA, 1980) Typical stressors likely to have set off the behavior that culminates in a transgression against the child are usually not to be considered as a failure to manage an emotional disturbance such as an active phobic state, a complaintive and compelling dread, nor the result of events characterized by hypervigilance, despite the fact that these disorders may have governed the child's formative years and over time moulded maladaptive traits. Nor is the essential intent of such a group capable of assisting a predominantly psychiatric population or one requiring desensitization therapy except as a modality perhaps for relaxation training for the autonomic physiologically affected. (Paul and Bernstein, 1973) For these adversely tension-controlled patients, referral to the appropriate systematic relieving psychiatrist is a must, probably in conjunction with a well monitored medication regimen. The social work therapeutic milieu lacks the conducive completion of hierarchal tasks to be effective and thus appropriate orientation is primary. Aaron T. Beck, 1976, who discusses the seemingly insurmountable fear that anxiety stricken patients display when fearful of confrontation or ill quips are rendered within the context of socialization spells an evaluative criteria to be assessed for.

Likewise the schizophrenic will not be able to follow normally held logic in order to participate productively. Oddities of thinking, depersonalization, irrational responses will stifle a group's give-and-take rational intuition and education often to a point of stopping any process in midstream. However as Jay Haley points out the need to identify in the attachment disordered syndromes one may be exposed to during childhood or adolescence, it may be helpful for patients to discuss inconsistencies of a parent in positively responding to the child's need for affection. My graduate instructor professor Thomas Szasz posed a much less radical concept for mental illness describing much psychiatric definition as controversial without agreed upon constructs. In his mental health bible The *Myth of Mental Health* he states there is no anatomical finding of mental illness in the postmortem. The discovery of self does not constitute a legitimate expectation for a return to normalcy for the illness of schizophrenia. Whereas clinical depression absents the individual from participation, either cautious or non disruptive, the issue of separation anxiety as it represents a disruption of bonding between parent and child must be addressed early on in most situations involving removal of the child from an abusive or neglectful and/or involving placement out of the home. (Grinker, 1966)

It is a far cry from the bulwark of theoreticians who prescribe predominantly for a population beseiged by pervasive difficult-to-treat symptomatology. The success of the group centered group as originally developed for a teacher population by Kemp, 1964, relies on what is in essence a Laing orientation, a framework which supports a belief that there are people who exhibit danger to self and others, who ought to be locked up. Despite the widespread belief that mental illness results from social deviation is supported by humanists such as Szasz, 1963, Bandura, 1968, and Phillips, 1968, the last two who claim that in technologically absent societies forms of psychosis are to be regarded as normal because the overall population is immature, the reality remains asserted to that in order to learn to confront one's inner confusion and turmoil one can best do so in a setting that permits a wide range of normalcy of social interaction.

Kemp developed his model for enhancing social interaction from primary and secondary school populations of the mid sixties basing his research on recitivism statistics. Patterns of group cohesion and honesty of participants line up with Bradford who lists group standards, climate which reduces anxiety and defensiveness, and defines involvement for retention of learning and stresses the positive significance of interpersonal transactions. Bradford is alone in his description as to the dynamics by which learning and problem solving occur in the class once fear and uncertainty arises. Kemp calls his article on "The Democratic Classroom" a method for improving the decision making process, freeing teaching staff from an autocratic orientation and reinforcing the actual learning process with a format that encourages psychological growth and dignity in the child groupings. The notion of a democratic foundation for cooperative decision making was new in its era, supported by Hopkins as to ways to improve the process by which instruction could best induce learning for the gradual confidence and ease of communication in order for the usual difficulty experienced by children who may be slow learners, by Kelley and Thibout who discuss group norms, planning for the classroom and goal setting and the type of participation likely to result in fulfillment of objectives.

The medical model of group therapy rests with treatment of

"pathos," with a perception of loss of significance in response to trauma as a personal methodology for coping with "emptiness." Adler, 1961, categorizes this "angst" or agony of the heart as merely a symptom of maladaptation. For some depressive patients, he agrees with Abraham, 1968, whose noteworthy definition of melancholia is based upon the severity of conflict combined with ambivalence. Abraham defines the integral concern of hostility as frustrated depression turned against the Self. Frequency of domestic disputes which involve violence produce a batterer who usually has a thought disorder often coupled with serious addiction and a spousal victim who may present with symptoms of depression or helplessness. Many psychoanalysts view depression in abused children as a hallmark of suffering brought on by a parent's inability to provide enough affection. The group as a system is aimed at correcting fallacies of thinking, at increasing self-esteem such that the participant can make healthier choices, and to help a person cope with less dependence on a perpetrator.

The most productive mechanism for eliciting positive regard within a group derives from having each group member describe their life story over a period of several months. Prevention occurs with education. (Block, 1967) The gradual process of redefinition does depend upon continual, consistent exposure to a learning process that has at its locus the instructive features for improved coping and increased tolerance, especially over issues of concern about actual control one has over their personal situation. (Koretsky, 1990) A several-month-long program of demystification as to family dynamics which may stem from one's family upbringing defines similarities that members can associate to regarding the chaos in the family and a resulting self image accompanied by internalized self messages and process for looking at repressed traits. Additionally a group's success at joining, providing empowerment, esteem and leadership introduce opportunities to restore painful emotional memories while also granting psychic space for breaking out of learned suppression of topics. As friendships and attachment occur within the group, participants are able to compare their value of experiences with a standard that is free of the armour dictated by a family code of false self ethics.

On the subject of relating the issue of the mother/child attachment becomes central to the often mentally carried image of the psuedo-mother, as posed by husband-wife team McCord and McCord, 1960. The need for a sense of commonality, community or belonging is viewed as one of the strongest values to ward off isolation and emotional numbing. The McCords define the self image that results from a rejecting, demanding, abusive parent as an adult child who has learned to suppress natural instinct, to squelch curiosity and creativity, to fit into rigid roles, follow a code of behavior that is often destructive, if not a facade, and in many ways shutdown attempts to be different through substance abuse, deviancy, destructive acts or suicide.

The pseudo-mother frustrates the child's desire to form a loving close relationship. Presumably this degree of thwarting exists because the psuedo-mother lacks a willingness to parent and be responsible to the act of providing for the minor's needs. In a world in which parents do their best and fail to provide "a minimum adequate standard of care and supervision" (Child Welfare Laws, 2000), the parent may be viewed as one who relies upon an instrument of corporal punishment or who is beleaguered by problems of her own and thereby unable to give the time or nurturing out of fear, intimidation, or phobia. The accepted postulate takes into account that a parent put in continual fear by a violent spouse cannot step beyond the confines of her relational limitation without engendering the hostility of the spouse. A parent who is under the continual shadow of substance abuse may not respond in a timely manner or at all when her child requires feeding or meals, bathing, dressing, transportation to and from school, or basic custodial care. Also, a parent too preoccupied by their own obsessions or depression cannot lift their head to look beyond their concerns to set those aside.

This author believes that the task of narcissism is to provide the child Self with an independent mirror separate from the acknowledged distortions of the parent. Into this identity go the idealized perceptions thereby psychologically freeing the adult from a destructive negating parent who does not appear to want to love and who puts the child on hold indefinitely for emotional attentiveness. Masterson, 1989, describes narcissists who are indelibly stuck in their self perceptions of an essential wound, who are openly aware of their continual need to receive attention, who without the desired attention become angry, bullying, and coercive to their detriment. Such an individual is often in their thirties and proceeds with a poorly adjusted coping mechanism in fending off stress, isolation, feelings of abandonment and feelings of inescapable sorrow for who they could have become were the intrapsychic wound less pervasive. Existential psychotherapists propose that this belief of sorrow for the psychologically injured Self can be somewhat offset by helping the patient view his or her experiences as real and making a commitment to their discovery of Self. (Heidigger,1962; May, 1967) The commitment to a search for meaning helps this type of individual work through issues of immediacy such as job dissatisfaction, relationships and personal safety in favor of evaluating larger life questions regarding death, personal metaphor and seeking experiences that give one significance. (Frankel, 1967) As the narcissist tests the transference as a new flight from falsehood and explores more devastating concerns of feeling devalued, he or she develops gradually a coping mechanism to ward off a sense of impending doom. The concern of guilt does not necessarily reflect criminal activity but connotes a belief of having survived tragedy or what could have been tragic. (Fromm, 1963)

The borderline personality disordered patient suffers from lack of meaning and depression by sinking into a feeling state, a bottomless pit, another type of negation of Self characterized by perceptions of personal emptiness. "I am bad," becomes a personal label, a discreet way to define the jagged edge of walking on too high a ledge or precipice. Without being paranoid, lacking persecutory delusions, the borderline is daily struck by their need to be so different from others they succeed in alienating the very people whose admiration they want. Both are mirrors to the soul, says Koretsky who thinks they can alter their basic orientation most of the time. Their aggressive tendency to lash out or pick at the value they perceive of in the counselor stands as a mirror for the slights and humiliations they have shored up over the years, despite their obvious intelligence, personal flair, creativity, and oddly their resources. Despite their attributes they rail against being incorrectly perceived, yet often have committed outrageous acts. (Laing, 1965)

Incorporated into this personal objective to free the Self from psychically crippling attachments, to see oneself as psychologically liberated (Fromm, 1963) is rewarded by the group process. Unveiling oneself through honesty becomes a powerful instrument with which to define any participation; the replacement of a pseudo-Self is only excepted by crisis therapy. (Albee, 1974) The degree to which the individual, parent or child, is able to honestly describe the traumatic events, the more they own it the truth of it resonates from within.

A very useful book that I found helpful for conceptualizing how group work ought to fulfill objectives is Virginia Satir's *Peoplemaking*. The other book that comprehensively explains the mother/child attachment and maturational development of the young child is Althea J. Horner's book on object relations. Another resource that tells of women's anger through their stories about personal crises is a one-time friend Dr. Harriet Goldhor Lerner who wrote *The Dance of Anger* on intimacy.

Because the use of metaphor is such a convincing anti-invective the cultivation of it is a legitimate focus. However most participants in a group will usually be self critical to a fault taking themselves too seriously and firmly unable to engage in the art of humor. Without humor sadly none progress past a harsh self critic which raises standards for perfection on impossible criterion. Metaphor is a soft method to nudge people past their internalized self fashioned critic which in seeking absence from chaos, inconsistency and abheration try to impose rigidity because it can be easily attached to for psychosocial needs of permanence. Many are already drawn to various metaphors through novels, ie escape from an overly industrialized city as in any of James Joyce's stories, the sense that trauma causes one to be stigmatized as in Nathaniel Hawthorne, the idea that one often discards the best of one's creativity in order to safeguard information and hide it from unwanted prying attention as in Guy de Maupassant's famous story. Movies also give us that ethereal identification with eternal allegory and imaging as in Anthony Hopkins' movies of Hannibal Lecter, a connivingly evil man who despite the best stings slips through every effort to contain him and gets his come-uppance anyways, Glenda Jackson as an unsatsified housewife whose husband falls in love with his closest friend in DH Lawrence's provocative story of death in a mine in Sons and Lovers, Glenn Close's flirtation and downfall for her fatal flaw in a torrid love affair from which she cannot recouperate her identity, and Helen Mirren's exacting character of a female lieutendant who stops at nothing until she apprehends a heinous killer. All these highly publicized ironies mould our society for the problems of the day giving us powerful instruments by which to measure our inclinations.

However without these spellbinding themes we must dig deep into our personal reservoirs to find resonating themes that can steer us as a guiding light of faith through hard times. Depending upon how well one knows oneself, the themes capable of becoming the fallback position when the threat of violence has seized one's life are the best advised. Traditional themes which offer resonance typically involve good and evil, search for truth, discovery that personal empowerment lies within, great achievements can be accomplished with persistent gradual study, a course of miracles opens the world to the awe-inspiring if one is in earnest with oneself and others. Humanistic psychology offers a spring board from which to satisfactorily palpate these realisms. Erick Fromm gave us a concept of self renewal based upon an individual's capacity for love, he states that by conquering narcissistic tendencies, the searching individual is able to assert over a fundamental urge to destroy.

Writing and art

I have over twenty years developed my own style for practice of treatment with regard to social work. Education in this career field relies almost entirely on theory. Those theoreticians whose works I have consulted tend to base their works on psychiatric patient treatment. Putting into practice the weekly treatment needed to guide the direction of a case requires being knowledgeable of theory and practice. My own work with adult children of alcoholics was stymied by a lack of literature that describes how to run a group. Yalom's bible on group psychotherapy while concerned with structure was not met by what I observed as a new practitioner. Thus when my publisher Dr. Erickson offered me a book contract back in 1987 I had by that date selected a criteria that combined generally agreed upon theory with the groups I was then leading. These consisted of education as well as clinical therapy groups for teen mothers (three per week for a year attended each by ten to twelve females), for adult alcoholics (two a week for four and a half years, some with five participants, others with an average attendance of twelve women, some groups that went almost two years) and groups led at high schools. Of approximately some forty men who attended numerous groups, approximately half had already served jail time.

By the time I entered social work I was expected to hang my own shingle. However I believed that whereas well-to-do upper middle class clients would inevitably drift toward other special interest groups such as bulimia, anxiety, professional training and the like, my skills could be best utilized by people with limited resources. Therefore I took a position inside a public welfare office seeing approximately thirty to forty child clients a year and their families. In this milieu I found most of my associates lacked masters degrees, almost all had no clinical experience and their contributions to the health of families was sorely unkind. I determined early that my training offered these families the best potential for recovery from very serious addictions, often coupled with severe violence and most, if not all, contained social groupings of narcissistic and borderline tempramentally dysfunctional parents. Because a social worker is expected to remedy the individual for whom allegations are written, he or she must be clear as to the level of disturbance and be knowledgeable of intervention practice. Thus the other successful coworkers were also therapists like myself with an average of five years work experience in agencies.

The literature produced by Social Work Journal (1975) describes public social welfare for child abuse as the necessary intervention on the child's behalf to protect the physical safety or keep the psychological intrapsychic boundaries of the child from emotional harm or neglect. This journal places discussion within the sector of public health. It provides studies that seek to prove the efficacy of social work as a methodology of research-governed principles that facilitate an understanding of the child's well-being. The emphasis is on what works. The populations studied fall within categories by age and type of institution according to public health issues.

The subjects of loss of attachment, lack of empathy, age appropriate expectations of the child by the parent, psychological safety from the perpetrator and parental self transparency form the foundation of child abuse treatment. Without a clinical awareness of how the child is affected for trauma recovery the average social worker cannot adequately assess for the impact of trauma. In order to be safe the child needs a program that speaks to her safety from emotional intrusion, from boundary and personal rights invasiveness, and from actual threat.

Issues of accountability get lost without a strategic well structured therapeutic intervention. Psychologists Margaret Mahler and Althea Horner subscribe to a belief that parent/child bonding is learned because the child carries a picture of the mother's loving. This introject becomes the degree to which the child is capable of passing through necessary milestones of individuation. Without the parent's ability to allow the child to be reassurred or soothed, the child does not perceive the world as safe. A child who cannot individuate often becomes personality disordered. This then becomes the method of discernment as to when the parent's behavior is unhealthy for the child. Social work as it has been historically regarded is given no emphasis for clinical therapeutic knowledge. Most social workers will say their training on the job only minimally prepares them to ask questions but does not give them enough theoretical comprehension to treat, even where a therapist already seeing the family does not understand what must be done to change the parent's behaviors that pose risk.

Satir (1983) takes the family as an entire grouping in order to make visible to the family the role of their identified patient, usually the child. In situations in which a psychiatric parent has allegedly placed a minor at risk, the assessment consists of evaluating whether that parent can safely provide for the child. Her style for interviewing is to interview an entire extended or blended family several times during the life of a case. She normalizes contact simply by discussing how each member views any family attitude, secret or role. This outcome is produced over ten to twenty sessions. The risk is framed within the context of that behavior that placed the child in harm's way and resolution grapples with two objectives primarily, achieving insight and changing the detrimental behavior in a fundamental result that decreases or eliminates risk to the child.

Kemp (1964) was the pioneer to examine ways in which what he calls a group centered group could accomplish similar expectations for all group members. His emphasis was for the educational system. He discusses various dynamics, psychosocial in nature, that may deflect from what was then a strictly psychoanalytic basis for psychiatric patients.

This theoretician poses that for special interests this type of milieu could bring about demystification as to the perception of social isolation. His model utilizes a traditionally psychoanalytic leader yet puts the tasks of ideaology as questions to the group. Thus groups must rely on a combined knowledge of such literature because whereas these psychologists have written information about the issue they do not instruct the practitioner in how this work can be done within the therapeutic setting. Only Koretsky (1990) tells how to keep the group centered as a group, formulate its own therapeutic milestones, teach tolerance and help participants to personally wrestle with their ambivalence. The group is kept to its focus by the skill of the therapist alone. This is possible solely with an orientation to group work which as it proceeds the trained therapist allows the group to redefine its roles for leadership. Autonomy then becomes its own identity.

Exacting as this work encompasses the formerly rigid structure of give and take, the therapist manuevers each member to exercise waiting to speak, offering compassion and a host of other aspects of tolerance until the group provides this focus for itself.

The law for child abuse concerns itself with the following:

(a) physical abuse
(b) neglect
(c) serious emotional abuse
(d) sexual abuse
(e) child is under five years of age and has suffered physical abuse by the parent, guardian or other such adult in charge of child's custody and supervision
(f) child's parent or guardian has been convicted of a death of another child through abuse or neglect
(g) abandonment
(h) the child has been freed for adoption from one or both parents for 12 months
(i) the child has been subjected to one or more acts of cruelty
(j) the child's sibling has been abused or neglected

After the petition is found to be true and a finding of disposition has been made in the county the child then is made a dependent of the court. The child then can be placed by edict either in the home in care of one or both parents or can be placed by order out of the home.

During this period defined as twelve months after disposition usually both parent(s) and child must receive services. Often there is an order for a case plan consisting of, but not limited to: counseling either together or apart, a parenting class, an Indivdual Educatioonal Plan for the child for a special educational program, visitation either supervised by an adult approved by the social worker or unsupervised, and regular frequent interviews with the social worker. The task of the social worker is to attempt to ameliorate the circumstances of risk to the child, present proof to the judge that the risk will not reoccur, and if separated reunite the child with a parent or ask the court to terminate parental rights and set the child free for adoption once the agency has identified an adoptive home.

The social worker is expected to do almost whatever is necessary in order to facilitate this process including counsel the parent and child to assess whether any age appropriate empathy exists. It is believed by many in this field that the minimally monthly face to face interview with the parent must incorporate the parent's agreement as to why they were charged. The parent must decide in what ways to conform. The social worker has but to meet, make the assessments and derive the course of action. In most service agencies the social worker has graduated high school, transferred by promotion and in rare circumstances has a Master's Degree with some practical experience in counseling patients. The work often demands an understanding of clinical outcome. A knowledge of each stage of change gives an experienced practitioner the spit and glue to decisively assist both parent and child toward the necessary outcomes.

Rage, feelings of personal emptiness and shame characterize an ever growing population. Masterson (1992) discusses borderline and narcissism as rage essential tasks of a disorder of attachment. Because these personality disorders result from a preoccupation that the emotional context lacks a fundamental support for that individual parent, the task is to bring about an awareness as to management of the aspects that are out of control. The general school of thought reflective of therapy is that these parents cannot parent. They are already too unpredictable in the way they respond to their environment, made this way by a perception they were so unloved that they were unable to inculcate into their gradual maturation any ability to separate themselves from others, or see themselves as separate.

In the patient population these adults have not been able to learn basic ways to interact without attempting to inflict emotional damage on others. The social worker without this orientation easily gets drawn into the chaos that borderline and narcissistic clients invite. The boundaries that contain these clients must be a principled structure consisting of regular therapy times, same day of the week, fees, and then keeping to a plan that takes that client past blame to explore issues of upbringing, trust, control over others, past therapy, personal and career goals, and agreeing to a lifestyle that gives the individual the least complication in day to day interactions.

Couples, never on their own to live alone, or develop apart from home and therefore own their psychological independence, when acquired of habitual chemical dependency use, begin to demonstrate patterns and atrophy of interests. Peele describes an internal symbiosis out of homeostasis, wherein withdrawal can cause illness, and tolerance increases an ability to adapt to drugs, both which threaten personal autonomy. Once autonomy is threatened it becomes more likely to suppress expression of personal assertiveness. R.D. Laing describes this profound negation as the individual is so detached he cannot get a sense of himself as an integrated being. In Science 1967 LSD was found to have caused genetic changes in chromosomes. The psychic dependency that occurs in the continual presence of a lover sees inhibition of reflexes and sensitivity to outside stimulation. For those for whom the relationship is like drugs, "life is a burden of useless struggles" drugs relieve. "They evade, mask or postpone the expression of needs and decisions." (Charles Winnick)

As with couples, the reason adolescents start drugs often is the result of fatalistic beliefs – the elixir resolves emptiness, where one is emotionally detached from people, has a restricted outlook, is passive, has not resolved childhood conflicts about personal autonomy and dependence. Attachment lessens an ability to deal with others or self and is increased dependency on the lover as the only source of reliance. Pessimism, anxious to face fears, dreads re-exposure, the cycle creates helplessness with an attending loss of discrimination and with this loss life is reduced to safe routines, a desire to stagnate and be untouched, for the "intoxicating effects" of drugs. Thus, drug dependent babies, hyper Ritalin children.

It is normal to take risks, risk-taking does not limit, or lessen, a person's capacity to live, or affect the quality of experience.

With non addiction one can do something because it brings joy to oneself. The goal is to work toward the sufficiency that permits one to live with an acceptance of uncertainty about our very existence.

Nathaniel Brandon poses an essential question for healthy functioning. He asks, "How does a person arrive at the state of being disconnected from his own emotional experience, of being unable to feel what things mean to him?" He begins his discussion as many addiction theorists do by stating, "To begin with, many parents teach children to repress their feelings. A little boy falls and hurts himself and is told sternly by his father, 'Men don't cry.' (p. 7) Emotionally remote and inhibited parents tend to produce emotionally remote and inhibited children – not only by the parent's overt communication but also by the example they set." It may be deduced that failure of self-acceptance leads a pre-adolescent into a quasi state of criminality. Thus, in a reference to his earlier work, The Psychology of Self-Esteem, Brandon says, "The nature of his self-evaluation has profound effects on a man's thinking processes, emotions, desires, values and goals." In this work he goes on to find "one of the tragedies of human development is that many of a person's most self-destructive acts are prompted by a blind, misguided (and subconscious) attempt to protect his sense of self ... when a person represses certain of his desires, because he cannot tolerate the anxiety of wondering whether he will attain them, an anxiety that makes him feel helpless and ineffectual, he disowns a part of himself." (p. 71) The Self is predominantly the Mind – "the client learns, not to assume responsibility for his life, but rather to recognize that he is responsible for his life." Brandon describes passivity as "when a person clings to the pain and frustration of childhood, refusing to see or move beyond it, he avoids awareness." (p. 83)

In *The Observing Self* author Arthur Deikman confirms the basic task of the therapy for the client is to "relieve psychological distress." (p. 97) The problem of purpose, not as an attempt to escape fear, helplessness or despair, is at the central existential questioning as health becomes restricted. He cites Maslow's intrinsic 'being' values and Wyatt's concerns for 'conduct' disorders.

The normative process of development for a child age 18 month (p. 69) involves picking up objects and tracking, whereas for the three year old experience is an awareness of awareness. The four to seven year old grows cognizant of learning to recognize relational differences and boundaries, and by eight years can relieve psychological distress (p. 97). The pre-adolescent finds a reciprocity of Self for healthy functioning reduces the intensity of affect (p. 110) as he moves away from being self-centered (p.117, 118) into a state of awake vs. a "hypnotic trance" of doing what others think he should. Thus Deikman provides a treatment for diminishing the anxiety that accompanies the corresponding functions of entry into youth for anxiety, depression, loss of interest in life, loss of self-esteem and hospitalization.

Charles Whitfield holds that the journey from a withholding or false self to an authentic self encompasses a fear of being exposed as a result of focusing on what others want, rather than on a hierarchy of human needs, mirroring for attention, loyalty and trust, (p. 20), the concept of the unfulfilled parent (pp. 21,22).

Well Health and Positive Esteem

Without trauma and ongoing emotional erosion of character, the normal child is cheerful, playful, respectful, observant and cautious as need be, depending upon his environment and the people with whom he interacts. He can sit through eight hours of school, engage with peers, run track and play an instrument in symphony. His years of education have fortified him with a repertoire of skills, reading, writing, story telling, puppet making, arithmetic, inventory counting, fractions, science, social studies, populations, cities, geography, geology, climates, desert, mountains, music, drama, and so on. His pleasure and enjoyment he takes in having mastered these subjects and his interest in himself and in others are the aspects that give him a positive outlook for his life.

The Petitions

Johnathan James

The petition reads, 'On or about September 3rd, 2008, the custodial parent was found to be intoxicated as evidenced by –
(a) the presence of empty liquor bottles lying on the floor numbering over twenty,
(b) a stale odor on Mrs. R's breath,
(c) an inability to be aroused by Pittsburg Police who entered the home,
(d) a test for substance that was read as positive for alcohol by the Pittsburg Health Department lab.

On said date the minor, under age 3, was found to have a severe diaper rash and to be in urine-drenched diapers. The minor appeared hungry, and there was no baby formula or food in the home."

On September 4th, 2008 during a hearing the judge made a finding for jurisdiction of neglect under a 300(b) on the basis that the arresting officer gave testimony as to the condition of the home. Also the physician on duty at the county hospital gave testimony that the minor seemed dehydrated and could have died. The health department lab test was entered as evidence. The judge made a finding as to the parent and ordered the minor be placed out of the home in a licensed foster care home.

On September 10, 2008 a hearing for disposition was heard. The petition was amended to include –

"The father's whereabouts is unknown."

The court ordered continued placement for the minor, a search for the father be begun, and services for the mother. The mother's case plan asks that she enter a substance abuse treatment program for a minimum of 90 days as approved by the county, that once she is completed she substance test weekly with negative results for a minimum of 6 months, and that she enter and complete a satisfactory residential program with the minor under a reunification plan.

Counsel was assigned as to the minor and the father respectively.

A home study for a suitable fost-adopt home was ordered if mother was unable to complete her 90 day program.

Family Law Status

This is the only marriage. The parents are legally separated.

Criminal history

Mrs. R has a federal index number for a conviction of being in possession of a controlled substance while driving a vehicle in 1991. A bench warrant was issued and she served time at a state penitentiary.

Psychological assessment

Mrs. R. is the youngest of three daughters raised by a disciplinarian military officer who restricted their activities in their adolescence. As a youth Mrs. R. was gifted academically with high grades and science honors. She received a scholarship to a private high school where she was entered into a junior academy for scientists. In her first two years there she worked with a faculty on uses of geology to study rock formations in desert environments. She published a paper on the use of marine pools in desert and received an honorable mention. When her youngest sister was school age her parents brought her home to help out with family duties. These absorbed her focus and by her final year her grades had fallen making her ineligible to enter a private college in Holland.

Standard high school achievement placed her with high scores. She received 790 in math and 780 in English. Her IQ was rated high, at 134. Her emotional quotient however was below age acceptability, thus necessitating further testing. She was given a Rorshach which rated her as having minimum psychological disturbance. Her MMPI showed her to be rigid and controlling with a predisposition for general subjects that vary minimally. Draw-A-Person showed the need for identifiers to be grouped in order for her to demonstrate proficient understanding.

Mrs. R. has received psychotherapy since age 20, when she suffered a dysporic mood adjustment around the time her younger sister was admitted to UC. She was prescribed Xanthrax and put on half-time work for six months. At age 27 she described feeling the world was too hard and she was feeling immense pressure to finish her doctorate. She was diagnosed with mood disorder and put on medication. When she was 32 she completed her doctorate and began working at a private mental health clinic seeing her own caseload of twenty patients. The following year she married. Her husband was a counselor where she worked. When she became pregnant she stopped working.

At this time attention is below average. She has a difficult time examining stress. Even before she gets to the end of discussion about stressors, she has begun focusing on another unrelated subject. It is a concern as to whether she can adequately anticipate the minor's needs, if she recognizes his cues and whether she will respond.

Dx 303.91 Severe Alcohol Dependence, Continuous
309.0   Dysthymic Mood Disorder

Current family situation

Mrs. R. was married in 2006 and legally separated in 2007 after the birth of her newborn. She presents as listless, dejected, depressed, self-medicating despite receiving medical monitoring. She describes the needs of her two year old as too difficult to handle and asked that the minor be placed temporarily until she can get back on her feet. Extended family live in another city; her mother's sister said she would come up for a few weeks to help Mrs. R. get on a routine. After the police entered her home and found her severely intoxicated they placed her under a 5150 hold to an emergency psychiatric ward at County hospital. There, she was observed for 48 hours before being transferred to the ABC Facility as a dual diagnosis candidate. She has not tested positive for alcohol since being admitted to ABC. She is permitted to reside there ninety days before she can be admitted to the mother-child residential county-run program.

The psychiatrist at ABC recommended Mrs. R. for daily testing, 90 AA meetings in ninety days, a medical evaluation which is partly underway, a parenting class and therapy with the staff psychologist.

Evaluation of the Child

Johnathan James was seen at the county health clinic by pediatric specialist physician on September 11, 2008. ENT was examined. Child is believed to weigh in below average for age and is being put on a special iron formula diet. He was last seen by a PHN in the home and examined for hives and was prescribed antibiotics. The PHN instructed the mother to bring the minor back once a week over the next month, but Mrs. R. failed to do so.

Johnathan is not on target for cognitive and motor functions. At times he has a listless gaze and appears drowsy. He walks with an even gait, shows normal stranger wariness suggesting an inclination to bond with his mother, hearing is good; he can crawl, hitch, roll over, climb, put objects into a bin, understand when his name is called and respond, follow directions, eat finger food and use a sippy cup.

The PHN believes it would be beneficial to place the minor in a toddler stimulation program at a nursery care and for his mother to join him as soon as her physician feels she is ready.

Recommendations

1. Order the child be placed.
2. Order mother participate in a plan of reunification.
3. Find the child is a person described by W&I Code Section 300.

Lisa Jones

The petition reads, as to counts 300(b) and (d) of the Welfare & Institutions Code:

"On or about January 8, 2007 the minor child was sexually abused, and there was substantial risk that her siblings would be sexually abused by his or her parent or guardian or member of the child's household."

"The parent or guardian failed to protect the child adequately from sexual abuse and the parent or guardian knew or reasonably should have known that the child was in danger of sexual abuse."

The petition further alleges as to a 300(i) count:

"On or about January 8, 2007 the minor child was subjected to an act or acts of cruelty by the step parent or guardian of the child's household, as evidenced by the fact the step parent willfully and knowing serious injury might occur did tape the minor's mouth and bound the minor's hands behind her back and locked her in a narrow closet for two days and two nights.

"On or about December 4, 2006; October 10, 2006; and September 11th and 12th, 2006 the step father did lock the minor in a closet each occurrence lasting over ten hours.

"The mother failed to protect the minor adequately from the acts of cruelty, and the parent reasonably should have known the min or was in danger of being subjected to an act or acts of cruelty."

A 300(j) count pertaining to two younger siblings says,

"There is a substantial risk of detriment that the minor's siblings will be abused or neglected, as defined in subdivision 300 (b), (d), and (i)."

Psychosocial evaluation

The presenting problem is the sustained allegation that the stepfather, Mr. John Bates, both committed cruel acts to his stepdaughter Lisa as well as inappropriately touched her in a sexual manner by putting his hand under her nightgown while she was sleeping and fondling her breast.

    The parents, John and Abby, are Caucasian, ages 37 and 31 respectively. John is tall, with dark blond wavy hair, well dressed, greenish gray eyes, small boned, and his wife Abby is medium height, warm blond hair to her shoulders, casually attired in pastel silks often a light blue open collared blouse and an ankle length dark blue or light green skirt and sandals, dark blue eyes, moderate boned. They both work at his physician office where he is an internist and she is a bookkeeper and nurse aide. Their hours at the office are from 8:00 am to about 6:00 pm. A daycare specialist takes the children – Lisa, age 8, John Jr., age 7, and Robbie, age 5, from school and keep them until 6:30 pm when Abby picks them up.
    Their residence is located in a middle class, older, well established suburb that is central to shops and about five minutes away from the school. The house is two story, about 1200 square feet, three bedrooms, one which the two young boys share, two baths and a fenced-in swimming pool and basketball court. The master bedroom and Lisa's are adjoined by a large master bath.
    The two older children are the products of Abby's first marriage. Robbie is her son by John. They have been married a little over five years. This is a second marriage for Abby and a first for John. They report their initial meeting at their church PWP group (Parents without Partners) as love at first sight and have spent every minute together until Robbie entered school.
    John has a DUI on record for speeding while intoxicated. This occurred in March 2002 prior to their meeting. He says it was a one time occurrence and since then he has attended AA meetings weekly to maintain support for his sobriety. Mrs. Bates has no criminal history.

Neither has a mental health history.

Abby was tested by weekly random testing for a month with negative results. John is under court order to substance test for six months by weekly random method. To date he has taken twenty random tests, and his tests are negative.

He was referred for psychological testing to a psychologist with twenty-five years expertise in conducting interviews for testing. He was given a Rorshach, for which he scored medium to high for personality disturbance of ideological thought; a MMPI, on which he was rated as having rigid controls as to parenting; on the Draw-A-Person the picture was incomplete as to normal expectations of what men his age and background put in.

He was administered testing for pedophilia by a retired police detective who hooked him up to a lie detector while having him review pictures of children at play and nudity in the bathtub. For a scale of 0-5 he was rated at 2.

He was interviewed as to his self report. He described feeling better at relating to young children rather than to many adults. He said he thought his profession caused him to view adult males as potential medical difficulties. He thinks of male children as naturally spontaneous, of having heightened needs for acceptance and as requiring some type of sexual education as to their prepubescent needs. He stated that the incident with his step daughter occurred after he had to punish her because she had failed to follow his directions about doing a chore completely and he was trying to figure out how to get her to pay better attention to him. He said he was trying the same thing he saw his father do with his older stepsister. He knows his father was wrong to do what he did, and that he is wrong as well, but it was the way his father controlled the house and kept "all his girls" in line. He feels his wife abdicates a lot by staying at the office, sometimes as late as 8:00 pm or 9:00 pm to take care of billing, leaving the burden of getting the children their dinner, bathing and getting tucked in at night.

The psychologist recommended the following,
1. John reside out of the family home;
2. John enter weekly therapy with a licensed clinician for a

minimum of six months to be evaluated at six months;
3. He focus upon learning normative needs for psychological safety for his children;
4. He join a treatment group and successfully complete a molest module aimed at redefining anger, control, and hostility directed at young children;
5. He continue to substance test by random methodology; and
6. He take a basic and an advanced parenting class.

It is not uncommon for adult male perpetrators to describe their reasons for molestation of a child in the family as,

a. living in an isolated community in which it is hard to meet peers;
b. cannot find girls who will agree to have sex with them;
c. a decision to give the oldest girl her first sexual experience;
d. wanting a divorce and choosing to force the wife into one out of anger;
e. having to do the babysitting for a maturing teenager;
f. angry the maturing teenager is having sex prematurely; or
g. wanting to see what it's like to step over a family boundary taboo.

The act of molestation, unlike emotional or physical abuse which are often equated with punishment, is an act of hostility. The primary indicator for consideration is whether there is psychological and physical safety in the home.

Questions for pre-evaluation for the psychosocial assessment by the investigative social worker are as follows,

Child

Does the perpetrator have continued access to the home? Who is in the home?

Is the child safe in the home?

Is the mother supportive of the child, or is she protecting the perpetrator?

Perpetrator

Is he actively on drugs?
If so, what is the amount he uses per day? Per week?
Is he on an AFDC grant?
What amount of earnings does he contribute to the household?
What is his relationship to his spouse?
Do they have frequent sex?
Is he supportive or unfriendly toward her?
What are the arrangements for parenting?

Jack Smith

The petition citing a 300(a) count for physical abuse reads,

"The child has suffered, and there is substantial risk that the child will suffer, serious physical harm inflicted non-accidentally upon the child by the child's parent or guardian, as evidenced by:

a-1 On or about June 21st, 2008 the child Jack suffered bruises on the face, arms and buttocks after his parent struck him with a belt;

a-2 On or about August 8th, 2008 the child suffered fractures on the face when the parent struck him with an object rolling pin;

a-3 On or about November 1st, 2008 the child suffered bruises to the arms and chest when the parent struck him with his fists.

a-4 Both parents were under the influence of a controlled substance at the time of all occurrences."

An investigation of these circumstances revealed the following citations as to the mother,

2003 admitted self to detox for 3 days, then admitted to ABC Substance Abuse Clinic and left against staff advice after 45 days;

2004 admitted after 5150 for suicide attempt to hospital for 72 hours, transferred to ABC, patient got into an argument with staff after 10 days and left facility against physician advice;

2005 smashed vehicle in tree, minors in the backseat asleep, 5150 to county hospital, was transferred after 105 hours to private mental health clinic as dual diagnosis, released after 1 month stay to husband;

2006 cited for DUI, was jailed for 48 hours, admitted to detox and inpatient treatment at county ranch for women, was discharged after 60 days, entered AA and outpatient chemical dependency therapy for 90 days when she completed program;

2008 mother with minor in infant car seat in backseat when she rear ended another vehicle, charged with involuntary manslaughter and DUI, convicted and sentenced for a month; minor placed, returned to father under order, case vacated.

Father had one DUI with positive test for cocaine in 1990. He was charged.

The court accepted the information during the dispositional hearing and ordered the case plan as follows,

1. Parents are to enter residential treatment for substance abuse for no less than 120 days;
2. During their stays they are to enroll and complete DEUCE;
3. Upon satisfactory discharge they are to test by random sampling weekly approved by Agency;
4. Parents are to enter outpatient substance treatment for no less than 90 days with on-site testing arranged;
5. Visitation with minor must be supervised;
6. Psychological evaluations ordered at 120 days of sobriety.

It should be noted that in California the law does not permit adults to be legally detained unless they are arrested by a police officer. Thus if an accident is caused by the parent it is involuntary manslaughter to the child if they are in the car. Ideally the court will order a parent entering diversion to be hospitalized on a psychiatric ward.

Psychological Evaluation as to Father /Summary

Subject: Marvin Smith
Age: 54
Status: Married
Children: Jack, 11; George, 7; and Paul, 2

The father Mr. Smith was tested 20 times in 30 days. He tested positive for cocaine and alcohol 19 times.

He was interviewed weekly over 7 weeks. His on report of his substance use was that he "cannot make it without a sniff or booze;" he stated he prefers "marijuana, ecstacy and coke" for days when his wife cannot join him. He states Jack's talking back to him upsets him. He does not believe a child should cook for himself, fail to bring home his bike or forget his new jacket at a friend's. He feels the child is being permitted to be irresponsible.

Diagnosis:　　Axis I　305.61 Cocaine abuse
　　　　　　　　　　　303.91 Alcohol abuse
　　　　　　　Axis II　301.89 Personality Disorder, Atypical

Recommendation: Detain to state hospital for 60 days in a locked inpatient facility in a substance abuse treatment program.

Steven Adamson

age 9

The petition as to the minor states as to a 300(c) count,

"The child is suffering, or is at substantial risk of detriment of suffering, serious emotional damage evidenced by severe anxiety, depression, withdrawal, or untoward aggressive behavior toward self and others as a result of the conduct of the parent or guardian, as shown by,

c-1 The minor's stepfather calls his son 'his sorry excuse for a son,' 'sissy', 'dumb shit' on a daily basis and has been doing so for about six months;

c-2 The minor's stepfather has locked him in his room for long hours in excess of three hours daily;

c-3 The stepfather will not allow the minor to sit at the dinner table and makes him eat in his room;

c-4 The minor is given too harsh restrictions by the stepfather and the mother does not interfere;

c-5 The minor's natural father is incarcerated."

Psychosocial Evaluation

Child

The child Steven was tested for academic performance. Scores were low. His academic IQ placed him at 100 as compared with his initial scoring of 120 when he first was enrolled. His teacher states that in the last half year she has noticed a considerable difference in his performance – he has difficulty concentrating, cannot answer questions without apparent confusion, appears to wander in discussions and has a hard time sitting still. Whereas in the past he took tests well, he now does not remember how to multiply or take essay tests.

I met with Steven 3 times. At the first session, he was shy and reserved. He answered questions with one or two words but did not elaborate. I gave him Draw-A-Person which he left incomplete. During the second interview he had a difficult time sitting. He took an interest in the sand tray and spent about five minutes with two soldiers and a tank which he had run over and kill a soldier. I asked him to tell me a story about it. He said, "The man in the tank never gets out. He hates everyone. He'd like the soldier to go away forever. My real dad said someday I'd be a soldier just like him. He said all boys become soldiers." When I asked him if this is his feeling as to how he is treated by his new father, he became quiet and did not answer.

At the third interview I showed him five pictures and asked him to tell me a story about each. For the picture of a house he said the man who used to live there had a fight and was in jail. For the picture of a man with a boy, he said that was his dad and himself. For the picture of the woman with a boy, he said his mother walks him to school two blocks away. For the family picture, he said he misses his father. For the last picture of a girl and a boy, he said his new dad wishes he had a girl. We talked about this for as long as he could tolerate. He said his new dad told him he married his mother so she could have a man around. Steven said his mother wants John to do everything. She wants the car fixed, the fence repaired, new towels and new rugs, and she wants John to tell him how to behave. Steven said he can't be quiet enough for John, so John sends him to his room all the time.

Diagnosis: 313.00 Overanxious Disorder
V62.30 Academic Problem

Father

John West is a 28 year old Hispanic who grew up the youngest of eight children. He works as a machinist on an assembly. He has had this job for six years and takes home good pay, over $2,000 a month. He says of his own father that he was a Marine, was seldom home and left all child rearing to his mother unless he was at home. His dad's word was God.

He expects to raise Steven. His first wife Mary left him because he wanted their child to grow up in the Pentecostal religion, and Mary was a staunch Catholic. He said he has talked to Steven's mother Doris about the importance of child rearing. Doris left all matters regarding her son to her first husband Greg. Greg was in the Army and raised Steven to be up at six, fold his clothes, prepare his own breakfast and go to school. He says while he was dating Doris he thought Steven was a great kid but now that he's around him he feels Steven doesn't have proper manners.

John was tested 22 times in a 30 day period and tested negative. He is clean and sober. He was given a Rorschach, an MMPI and Draw-A-Person. Results ranked him as meticulous at details, overly concerned with appearances, and generally critical of people in his immediate surroundings.

Diagnosis: R/O Schizoid Personality Disorder, 301.20

Recommendation

1. Mr. West to complete a psychological evaluation.
2. Mrs. West to admit to a 90 day treatment facility that will permit her to reside with her son.
3. Upon satisfactory completion, Mrs. West to test random substance abuse for a minimum of six months with negative tests.
4. The couple to enter individual therapy to explore issues of alienation of the child, creative play, parent/child

communication, and psychological safety.
5. therapist approved by social worker to examine discipline and child rearing practices, and any other relevant issues of the spousal unit.

The Model for the Interviews

The social scientific foundation for assessment of psychosocial behavior is to be found in a standard grouping consisting of normative adults, thought ordered adults, adolescents, children and toddlers. Focus centers on distinguishing between normative thinking in parents and the subsequent impact of socialization on their children when normal systems break down. The initial assessment must include an evaluation of the health of the family unit and child and must address the following –

>   Behavior
>   Psychological isolation or futility
>   Attachment
>   Tolerance of complexity
>   Family structure of flexibility
>   Resources, financial and emotional

The evaluation takes about four to six face-to-face visits of one to two hours per visit to complete and is based almost entirely on observation. Observation includes raporte between parent and child, the child's response to crisis, his preparation for tasks, adaptive setting transitions and stranger wariness. These four to six interviews include both parents, where two exist, all children, and if it can be arranged the extended family. The first hour should be with the parent or parents about the allegations governing the situation; at least ten minutes to involve the child or children, and about a half hour with the child or with each child. Discussions with children should be light weight – about their school, classes they take, who teaches, which parent helps with assignments, who has met the principal, after-school activities, coaches, friends at school, friends at home, favorite color, TV program, last time the family went somewhere.

Further evaluation should discuss the thorough extent of parental capability, the parent's understanding of their child's needs, non corporal punishment, and any stressors that the family faces. In addition, reports may include medical history, immunizations, hospitalizations, psychological evaluations, substance abuse chronologies, Individual Education Progress notations from the school, psychosocial and academic testing and police reports.

Once these reports have been received and updated, the social work professional must assess for risk of detriment – specifically for physical safety in the home and for psychological safety of relationships. This assessment is comprised first and foremost of a hierarchy of concerns which typify safety for the child who is potentially at risk.

Is the child likely to be injured or killed if left in the current situation?
Is the child likely to suffer emotional damage if left in the situation?
Does the perpetrator have access to the child?
Do the parents protect?
Is there extended family to whom the child can confide?
Is the child old enough to seek out help?
Is the parent functioning at a basic level?
Is the parent's judgement impaired due to substance use,

mental illness or organic illness?

There will arise crises that require yet more one on one sessions. Many of these are medical. The social worker may have fragile infants who must be seen weekly and possibly daily until the medical problem becomes stable. These problems include pumping out the lungs, changing tubes in the ears for chronic ear infections, setting up intravenous feeds, strip testing for low glucose and maintaining a complex diet for a severely handicapped child. Such presentations may require weekly visits to the home for up to three months before the child can be seen every three weeks. In-home information may consist of checking equipment such as a respirator or EEG every two weeks to assure it is working. Also the social worker has to have in-depth discussion with the foster parent or nursing home with regard to meal times and ability of the baby to keep down liquid and/or food, age appropriate weight gain with consultation with physician, and child's crawling, motor skills, and seeing and hearing.

The federal government mandates there will be a minimum of one face-to-face contact with the family each month for one hour. Due to the prevailing severity of family dynamic of severe substance abuse coupled with a rejecting maternal figure or a combative spouse, the frequency and amount of contact has to become intensified. Thus, the recommended face-to-face contact is as follows:

For the first month, 4 sessions of one to two hours each with the parents over four weeks. During this initial evaluative work the social worker needs to identify a rejecting mother with an extreme failure to thrive indicated primarily by lack of any weight gain causing an infant to seem "light as air;" also to target the presence of depression, hostility, a mental health disorder, and anti-social loss of control due to drug and/or alcohol use.

Also in the first month, 4 sessions of approximately one-half hour face-to-face with the child at home and one to three one-half hour with the child either at his school with the principal or in his therapy to further assess consistency of his behavior in different settings.

For the second through the fourth month, face-to-face contact should be divided as follows: 2 sessions each month for two hours consisting of one hour with the parents, one-half hour with the parents and child, and one-half hour with the child alone.
After two to six sessions the social worker has made an initial evaluation as to family dynamic.

After the fourth month, there should be 1 session every three weeks for up to a year and possibly extending to eighteen months.

Each monthly or bi-weekly session should follow the following format: (a) delve into any discussion of relevance to the spousal unit including but not limited to spousal conflict, trust in the family, and interactions with the child; (b) look at progress made on the Case Plan; and (c) any feelings and ideas elicited through discussion and homework.

Crisis intervention for a parent/teen conflict may necessitate a four hour session to facilitate and re-enforce the rules of the home and smooth out essential misunderstandings.

At the end of six months visitation is evaluated for whether the family is ready to move from supervised to unsupervised contact. By this time, the parent or parents have to have demonstrated their ability to create psychological safety for the child.

At the end of a year the court usually ends the case by vacating dependency and terminating services.

This then is the model. Historically this type of interactive model is based upon a medical intervention addressed in the derived forms of youth, teen and parent guidance centers nationwide.

The following psychotherapists and educators initially introduced the two day intensive as an emergency intervention for when a teenager residing in the home assaulted a custodial parent. Medical assessment to determine if the teen needed sedation and observation for this tyrannical behavior required an overnight stay in a hospital setting. Some hundred years later the didactic hospital stay became utilized as institutes for parents who suffered from cancer, severe illness and severe loss of functioning to ease the knowledge of eventual trauma and loss for both parent and family, and to provide learning and mainstream education.

Carole W. Bowdry, MSSW, of the Tavistock Clinic in Texas wrote "Diagnosing the Severity of Physical Abuse as a Case Management Tool" for a training coursebook for the Texas Department of Human Resources that was utilized in coursework in California Risk Assessment Curriculum for Child Welfare Services. She defines high risk into several categories as follows.

(A) Severity and frequency of abuse was catalogued by emergency medical treatment or required hospitalization; abuse of a sibling that resulted in death or permanent loss of functioning of organs and limbs; serious injuries at different stages of healing; severe emotional harm and any sex abuse.

(B) Location of injury includes the head, face, neck, anus or genitals and internal organs.

(C) Pending allegations including previous serious substance abuse.

(D) Child's age and capabilities – can the child care for himself? Is he under age 5, delayed, or chronically ill?

(E) Is the perpetrator in the home with complete access to the child? Are there many perpetrators?

(F) Child/Caretaker interaction – is it characterized domestic violence, parental alienation, poor nurturing, inappropriate or excessive punishment, failure to recognize age appropriate behaviors and unrealistic expectations, does drug/alcohol treatment continue, and does the parent exhibit impaired judgement such that the child's environment of safety is compromised?

Dr. Lydia Rapoport, Associate Professor, School of Social Welfare at University of California, takes the viewpoint that crisis thwarts the child's normative responses to his environment. Crisis, she says, is a disaster, an environmental event which constitutes an external threat. The individual responds with symptoms of stress. It can be an event that strengthens one's capability to adapt, per W.I. Thomas. Dr. Gerald Caplan, Director of

Laboratory of Community Psychiatry at Harvard, calls crisis a continuing state of reacting to stress ie a death or loss. It is not an illness, but a threat to one's fundamental integrity or a state of acute deprivation, and met with depression. Energy needed to keep repression of unsolved problem, with therapy, may become available to solve the current problem.

There is impact, a period of recoiling, and a post traumatic period, says Dr. James S. Tyhurst, in his unpublished speech of "Role of Transition States – Including Disasters – in Mental Illness," at The Symposium on Preventive and Social Psychiatry, of Walter Reed Army Institute of Research, Washington, D.C., 1957. If habitual problem-solving fails, emergency problem-solving mechanisms are utilized, and avoidance of need-resignation begins or a state of major disorganization follows.

The Tavistock Clinic studied separate trauma of young children entering a hospital and found they experienced symptoms of protest, despair and detachment. In this last state defenses of the youngster become shallow attachments and being self-centered. An adult may respond with somatization or displacement. Therapy may require "rehearsal for reality." The social worker's task is to first clarify the problem with the goal of cognitive restructuring. The client may not be aware of the stressor. The social worker needs to help manage the emotional state, put experiences into a rational context, and then define support networks.

Agnes Ritchie, Chief Social Worker for the Division of Child Psychiatry at the University of Texas, states in her article "Multiple Impact Therapy," first published in Social Work, Vol. 5, No. 3, 1960, that the initial assessment of a family in crisis necessarily should be handled by a team. The team would ideally consist of a psychiatrist who sees the teen, a clinical psychologist for a second or third child, a psychiatric social worker for the mother and a resident clinical psychologist or intern who works with the father. This constitutes the standard arrangement for treatment practiced at the Youth Development Project at Galveston, Texas, in 1952, a service for teens and their families consisting of a two-day intensive by a team. She remarks that after an initial family-team conference, followed by individual interviews, joint interviews ought to be overlapping and as flexible a staffing pattern as will yield a willingness of family members to share insights. Psychological tests are given to the teen. On the second day the problem is discussed with recommendations and insights. Differences between team members are explored in the presence of family with no lack of mutual respect and with encouragement of the family to find answers on their own. There is very little history taking although relevant family history such as developmental history of the teen, history of conflicts in the family, rules and how they are changed gets discussed. The team approach tends to be useful for chronic runaways, delinquent acting-out, school failure, and sexual deviations, each which requires approximately fifty hours of interviews.

Elizabeth E. Irvine, Senior Caseworker at the Tavistock Clinic in Texas, teaches a course on casework. In her article "Children at Risk" published in Case Conference, Vol. 10, No. 10, 1964, she studies children of parents who were admitted to a mental hospital to examine the issue of vulnerable defenses for the youngster. She cogently summarizes risk for this population – as a child who experiences the sudden, although not necessarily permanent, loss of a parent, who enters into foster care or goes to live with a relative, and whose normal expression of a varietal range of emotion becomes stymied as a mask of indifference. The social worker's goal is to help the child deal with the inner crisis. Because children exposed to scenes of domestic violence may produce enuresis or encopresis, confusion for the child may evoke a lack of tolerance to his expression over grief and loss, unrealistic anxiety and guilt. The home may blame the child, parents may get jealous of foster parents, the child may refuse to go to school. Irvine cites two references – "A Unit for Mothers and Babies in a Psychiatric Hospital," from Journal of Child Psychology and Psychiatry, Vol. III, No. 1, 1962; and British Journal of Psychiatric Social Work, Vol. VII, No. 2, 1963.

Mordecai Kaffman, Psychiatrist-in-Chief, Child Clinic of Kibbutzim, Israel, in his article "Short-Term Family Therapy" evaluates seventy social work cases of children seen in a child guidance clinic. These child subjects were analyzed for the efficacy of short-term treatment for emotional disorders in acute situations leading to a breakdown in previously normal behaviors. Treatment focused on an integrated family interaction, conflicts between child and parent personalities, and reformulation of family dynamics. The intake interview was made up of key developments, medical history, traumatic events, and family relationships. The goal was to bring about a healthy family readjustment after a trauma and was accomplished within three months of treatment. During this three month period there were any combination of interviews, a focus on discussing shared insights as a methodology for coping with severe conflicts. Typical treatment per family consisted of meeting with the parents once, meeting with the child three times alone, meeting the child and the parents six times or more, and meeting the father once.

On the role of the family author Jerome Kagan in his book *The Nature of the Child* looks at a number of cultures – Java, Japan and China – in which the behaviors that produce necessary developmental milestones are examined for their seemingly undersocialized morales. The suppression of personal feelings occurs so as not to hurt others emotionally; incomplete toilet training at age three is viewed nevertheless in older years as a factor of aggression, although aggression as desirable in order to accomplish objectives is modeled by the social class as is autonomous choice, rejection of peers, the increase of cognitive growth, secure attachment and an inhibition of lying, destruction of property, stealing and combative verbal objections. The passive, dependent mother, without intellectual curiosity who is suspicious may arouse a physical fear of disapproval, and excessive restriction as a check on impulsivity may create self condemnation, antagonism and a personality prone to anger. Social displays of love versus restrictions, while meant to provide a choice of standards to adopt, formulate much of adolescent behavior, from truancy, emancipation, psychological freedom, private conscience, acceptance of role models, sense of worthiness and handling frustration.

Eclectic practitioners base their theory on observation, having formulated models of therapy outcomes on therapeutic goals for actualization. These vary from the medical model for which the aims are few – diminishment of symptoms of psychic illness and despair, rudimentary intervention with medication, and safety for withdrawal from drugs with hospitalization.

Treatment Problems

Treatment Plan of Daniel

Born, 1928
Education, Vienna, Austria

PRESENTATION
Enjoys European lifestyle
Close relationships with family, is married
Never does laundry, almost never eats in
Lives by upper middle class standard
Is not seen by most people who might have some interaction
Conflicted, seldom gets away from it

ASSESSMENT
Anxiety, limited self introject
Ability to discuss without attempts at deception
Enjoys primary relationships

TREATMENT
Must have self awareness of motivation

RECOMMENDATIONS
Identify and assess intolerance
Look for ambivalence of life
Obtain patient's self description of what separates him in his mind from others
Discuss when patient talks himself out of compromise
Instruct patient how to tolerate uncertainties

Family Case Plan for John

Born, 1970
Education, Venice, Italy

ASSESSMENT
Estranged from family of origin
Very good parent of son, married living apart
Easily angered, takes it out on perceived valued
persons of allied therapist
Resistant initially to acknowledged treatment

DIAGNOSTICS
Egocentric, reactive behavior
Personality disordered thinking, likes to show people up
Cavalier, defends against depression

TREATMENT
Needs to demonstrate awareness of depression

RECOMMENDATIONS
Must be able to sit with own emotional content
Must demonstrate willing self insight into need for destructive activities
Regular visitation with son

Family Case Plan for Paul

Born, 1938
Education, Venice, Italy

PRESENTATION
Affable, interacts well with others, concerned
Self definition secure, no personality disorder
Very good living structure, can vary
Knows own limits, exhibits contientious decision-making
Lives well, easily

ASSESSMENT
Interpersonal exploitation, lack of empathy
Ability to change one's behavior, unknown
Close to mother, despises father

TREATMENT
Develop limits
Determine honesty, rights of others
Provide patient with new family, new friends, new associates

RECOMMENDATIONS
Evaluate standard of ethics
Replace exploitation with empathy

Case Plan for Edward

Born, 1938
Education, Liverpool, England

PRESENTATION
Misanthropic sexual hatred toward female authorities
Grandiosity, thinks he has a right to usurp power
Interpersonal exploitation, lack of empathy, seeks to intimidate and control
Falsely engenders emotion while becoming professionally combative

ASSESSMENT
Histrionic personality disorder, mood sometimes dystonic
Flattened affect, irrationality, tantrums

TREATMENT
Develop empathy, ego syntonic objectivity, concern for rights of others

RECOMMENDATIONS
Develop greater self awareness, emotionally link maladaptive behaviors to negative outcomes
Develop strengths
Seek positive regard with men in sexual relationships

Case Plan for Adam

Born, 1932
Education, Naples, Italy

PRESENTATION
Knows the difference between right and wrong, refuses to do the right action
Is a self professed homosexual, might have HIV
Enjoys the company of females

ASSESSMENT
Narcissistic, ego syntonic
Identifies with the oppressor for personal power

TREATMENT
Self manage own tendedncies toward usurping authoritative power of others
Link emotions with appropriate behaviors
Encourage patient to become less domineering, judgemental
Teach patient to tolerate conflict, ambivalence

Reports on Ajudication

For Alcohol – 300(b) and (g):

"On or about January 17, 2003 the Superior Court upon finding abandonment by custodial parent Jonas Lafferty did award the minor LAURENCE LAFFERTY, age 7, and his two younger siblings, LUCIA GAVIN, age 6, and DELIA GAVIN, age 3, to the mother of Laurence, Melissa Lafferty under a protective order. The biological mother of the Gavin minors is deceased.

"On or about January 2, 2004, the mother Melissa Lafferty was found drunk and disorderly in Sanchez Park taking a bath in the public square fountain and asking strangers if they would like to buy DELIA GAVIN, age 3, and take her home.

"On or about January 2, 2004, the Police did arrest the minor's step-mother/guardian and detain her in county jail for 72 hours whereupon she was released to ABC Detoxification and Rehabilitation with the minor, DELIA.

"On or about January 2, 2004, the Police did find the minor LUCIA GAVIN, age 7, to have been left in the care of LAURENCE LAFFERTY, age 8, and by negligent failure to provide adequate food, clothing, shelter, medical treatment and custodial supervision, there is substantial risk the minors will suffer serious physical harm or illness.

"The inability of the biological father of the three minors, Jonas Lafferty, age 35, to provide regular care for the children is evidenced by the fact that he has not returned to their home nor contacted his ex-wife or his parents since January 17, 2003."

The LAFFERTY/GAVIN case was heard in Judge Rudolph Steiner's courtroom on January 7, 2002 as a result of the above petition being filed. Judge Steiner made a finding for disposition after he ascertained from the police that the mother was arrested on January 2, 2004 and was administered a substance test. The test was determined positive for alcohol and barbiturates and was entered as evidence. Also on January 2, 2004 Judge Steiner found the minor Delia to come under a 300(b) of the Welfare & Institutions Code and found the minors Laurence Lafferty and Lucia Gavin to come under Sections 300(g) and (b). Delia was ordered into rehabilitation with stepmother/guardian Melissa Lafferty.

An investigator familiar with the three minors stated under oath that after Ms. Loretta Gavin drowned in a boating accident in winter of 2002 the children spent week nights at the home of Melissa Lafferty and she drove them to their father's on weekends. The investigator said all children think of Melissa as their mother. Other pertinent information given the Superior Court is as follows: the parents' relationship has been close and supportive with Mr. Jonas Lafferty, father, paying child support and alimony since 2000 by his own request. The father has spent every Friday afternoon at Ms. Lafferty's home as part of their arrangement up to the 2003 incident when he left the children without care for an entire weekend when he took Melvina Gavin, age 22, to Tahoe on his motorcycle to elope. He has not returned to the home or gone to his job. Jonas Lafferty works for Isleton Factory, Inc. for the past twelve years where he takes home approximately $2,150 a month, pays out $975 in support, owns his home and has been considered stable and reliable. Mr. Lafferty has had an unusually close relationship to his dead wife's father and regards him as family. According to recorded contacts the senior Gavins are unable to provide custodial care for the minors whom they say Lucia was very close to her mother; they believe their son is on heavy drugs again.

The two older minors were seen in therapy on January 3rd, 2004, January 4th, 2004, and again on January 6th, 2004. The psychologist, Dr. Stella Ealy, concluded that Lucia is likely suffering from a traumatic attachment loss as a result of her father's abandonment. Laurence is displaying some acting-out behavior of bringing dirt into the home and leaving it on the coffee table with a straw. He said on one occasion his father gets high with his aunt. He also says Lucia's and Delia's mother began as his after school daycare provider. Dr. Ealy has recommended foster care for the two older minors with Laurence to enter a medical facility for thirty days prior to joining his sister Lucia.

Analysis: This is a fairly typical episode of abandonment due to substance abuse on the part of each parent. The father may be using cocaine or methamphetamine. Because he has not returned to his obligations nor made arrangements for custodial care, it can be assumed that he has abandoned his children. Up until now the mother has provided a stable environment for her son and two stepchildren. Her bout with alcohol places them at severe risk if she cannot curtail use. The treatment plan for her that is ordered is complete rehabilitation prior to re-entering society. It must also include frequent testing for at least a year, counseling twice a week, AA several times a week, and care of all children in her program. For father, if he returns and wants to become a custodial parent, he will have to test for substance abuse and if tests are positive, he must enter a year-long rehabilitation program to include frequent testing, group diversion, individual therapy, and parenting education.

For methamphetamines – 300(b) and (c):

"On or about September 28 of this year, the minors CATHERYN, age 4, and MARCUS, age 5, were detained in custody when the police discovered the following:

(1) the home was cluttered with household objects and stacks of newspapers from the floor to the ceiling preventing entry or walking;
(2) the garage and kitchen pantry smelled of rotten garbage and was so foul it was hard not to gag;
(3) there was no food in the refrigerator except baby food on the shelves and on the stove were pots containing cracked fluid;

(4) the youngest minor's bed was piled with bed linens and towels making it impossible to use for sleep; and
(5) inside the shed in the backyard there is a bed but no toilet facility or running water.

"The minors' parents CATHY and MARC STETTER were arrested for manufacturing methamphetamines in the residence of the minors."

A jurisdictional hearing was held the following day at 0900 hours in Superior Court in Department 1 of Judge Rudolph Steiner. The two police officers who conducted a raid and shut the home down for uninhabitable conditions were sworn in. Judge Steiner found in favor of jurisdiction. A date for disposition was set for two weeks.

At the disposition hearing both parents were present with attorneys. A contest date was set for a week to hear other evidence. However, the judge ordered a temporary stay for out-of-home placement.

At the contested disposition the court heard from the father's foreman that the father worked nights for the bridge and took home four grand a month. The landlord claimed under oath the family rented a three bedroom home for six years and was regular with rent. The mother's father showed the court receipts of work done that contradicted the length of time the house could have been in such a state under thirty days. The judge ruled that the minors were to become dependents under Section 300(b) and because of their age also (c) writing that "the child is suffering or is at substantial risk of suffering serious emotional damage evidenced by severe anxiety, depression, withdrawal or untoward aggressive behavior toward self or others because the child has no parent or guardian capable of providing appropriate care." He ordered out-of-home placement, ordered parents into drug rehabilitation and no visitation with minors for first ninety days. He asked the Social Services Department to locate a suitable relative for possible guardianship or adoption.

An investigation showed a paternal grandparent had sexually molested a cousin per section 11165.1 of the Penal Code. The mother had a sister, age 39, who resided in Belvedere on a houseboat with her husband. The mother's father agreed to accept custodial care only if his daughter could not raise the children but asked for a home to take them because he has to work long hours. The agency will seek a babysitter who can care for the two children at night while maternal grandfather is at work, so the minors can be placed in his custody.

Analysis: The long term problem for methamphetamine manufacture is the pay incentive. For thirty hours cooking a couple can earn $30,000 in cash. Some manufacturers do quite well. They cook several batches a year and pay a staff of two. The other difficulty is the mother's father does not view the problem quite the same, he thinks the barricade is for the manufacturing to keep the kids and neighbors out. At this point we would assume he knows the family probably better than anyone else although he may not know whether they are also drug users of the batches they cook.

For cocaine addiction – 300(d):

"On or about 2:00 am on the 19th of August the minor GERTRUDE states her stepfather came into her bedroom and watched her sleep.

"On or about midnight of the following Saturday night the minor states her stepfather came into her bedroom and lay on top of her.

"On or about August 27th of this year the minor told her mother that she did not feel safe around her stepfather and asked if she could live with a friend of hers from school to finish out her last year of high school.

"On or about August 30th of this year the mother requested her husband be drug tested. He tested positive for cocaine."

A jurisdictional hearing on September 2nd of this year found the events to be true as described. On September 12th of this year Judge Rudolph Steiner found that the minor was a dependent child described under section 300(d) and ordered the stepfather out of the home in drug treatment, ordered the mother and minor into therapy twice a week and if the therapist agreed, overnight visits at the home for the minor.

By the first six month hearing the mother had filed for divorce and put her house on the market for sale with plans to obtain a three bedroom condo in a gated area. The allegations were dropped but the case held open six months under a voluntary order.

For bizarre cruelty – 300(i):

"The child RADIA BENEFICIO, age 6, has been subjected to an act or acts of cruelty by the parent or a member of the child's household, in that:

(i-1) "On or about November 3rd of this year during a birthday party the minor's family put on strange wigs and wore odd costumes and struck her arms and legs with sticks and metallic objects;

(i-2) "On or about November 3rd of this year the mother of the minor RADIA, age 6, put lines of dye consisting of deep brown, red and off blue color on her daughter's face and the color cannot fade or be soaped off;

(i-3) "On or about November 3rd of this year the father of the minor RADIA became overwhelmed by her face paint and shaved her head; and

(i-4) "On or about November 3rd of this year the uncle of the minor RADIA murmured incantations over the minor's head and shook the minor hard enough for her to fall on the floor and sustain an injury."

On November 4th of this year the presiding judge said this was the worst case he had ever come across involving bizarre cruel and unusual behavior perpetrated against a small child. He made a finding simultaneously for jurisdiction and disposition for 300(i). Disposition was continued pending an order both the child be examined, the parents be detained and drug tested. Tests returned positive in large quantities for LSD, as to father, and methamphetamine, as to mother. An unknown substance found in specimen of mother was sent to a special lab for additional testing. The test showed X-enzyme, a little known drug which when taken in sufficient doseage results in hallucinations and distortions up to 105 hours. As a result of testing, the social therapist had filed a JV-180. A Modification Petition Attachment JV-180 of the Welfare & Institutions Code, 388, is filed to change the circumstances and modify the petition based upon new evidence.

On November 18th of this year the continued matter was turned over to Judge Rudolph Steiner who ordered parental rights be terminated, that the child be freed for adoption and that the department make a speedy search for an adoptive home.

Analysis: Parental rights are seldom terminated before parents have been granted every possible permission under the law. In this situation it is the unusual behavior that these parents have used permanent dye on their child's skin that removes their parental rights. The modification of law which must be accompanied by a 388 and a subsequent hearing is a fairly recent law, 1993 by the Judicial Court of California, and allows for a ruling to be set aside in favor of new evidence. In this matter the evidence of the test for hallucinogens is overwhelming as to repudiate accidental circumstance. Overriding conscientious objections to practicality as to parental logic in creating a safe social setting has to be regarded for each parent's state of mind at the time of their child's party.

For restraining order as a result of alcohol consumption – 300(e) and JV-250:

"The child MICHAEL is under the age of five and has suffered severe physical abuse by a parent or by any person known by the parent and the parent knew or reasonably should have known that the person was physically abusing the child, in that:

(e-1) "The parent Dr. James Idol, MD, while intoxicated under the influence of alcohol on or about December 10th at 0100 hours did batter the minor with rings on his bare hands until the minor's body bled;

(e-2) "The police apprehended Dr. James Idol charging and arresting him on or about December 10th of this year at 1345 hours on charges of willful malice and criminal negligence for hitting his son, the minor, severely to cause welts over his face and body;

(e-3) "County Hospital Dr. MacGregory, Pediatrics, examined the minor Michael on or about December 10th of this year at 1915 hours and described that the minor suffered over twenty welts each about one centimeter wide and a quarter to a half inch long, several bloodied, many bruised dark red and purplish, each painful to touch;

(e-4) "On or about December 10th of this year, nearly one and a half hours after the hitting ceased, the minor is alleged to have complained to his father who is reported to have yelled, 'If you say another word to me I will strike you like a rag on the ground," overheard by an officer of the law who witnessed the remark at Burger King; and

(e-5) "The minor's mother has not resided with the minor since the minor was two and her whereabouts are unknown."

After the minor was placed in foster care a JV-250 was filed forbidding the father to enter onto school grounds or going near the minor in public. The original petition was filed on December 11th of this year. A Jurisdiction hearing determined the events were true, and a Disposition hearing found the minor to be a dependent under section 300(e). In the dispositional hearing petitioner and counsel amended the petition on its face striking the words 'to have yelled... on the ground' and in their place, threatened with intimidation. In court the police officer who booked Dr. James Idol, MD, gave testimony that he substance tested Dr. Idol and that the test showed toxic levels of alcohol in his urine. The judge ordered father into residential rehabilitation for a minimum period of ninety days with treatment including frequent testing, group psychotherapy and individual counseling twice a week with a separate educational component on battery, and because he is a doctor of medicine, surgery, he was ordered into any program managed by physician staff. A case plan was ordered for the mother if she is found. The judge ordered a complete investigation into Dr. Idol's history.

A continued investigation revealed documentation in other states. Dr. Idol was arraigned but not convicted in the state of Florida for battery of a spouse in which he roughed her up causing dark outlines around the tip of each finger beneath the nails to form. In Wyoming charges were filed against Dr. Idol for battery of a Latino nurse during an argument which led to her receiving a thrombosis line of discoloration to the neck. Dr. Idol was arraigned but due to insufficient evidence he was not convicted. He was given credit for 45 days in jail without bond.

Analysis: Dr. James Idol, M.D., is a surgeon who during an operation regulates the pump. He is assigned with watching REM, counting absorption to blood by intravenous and monitoring the cardiogram scope, and assessing for signs of acute thrombosis. His medicine practice gives him peculiar types of information which must figure in what he decides to use as domestic violence on a spouse since both outcomes can only be produced if the spouse is either imbibing liquid or ranting. Because he has a criminal record, he is to be considered dangerous. Severe injury of a minor under age five restricts visitation and places the adult squarely in the realm of narcissistic impulsivity and lays the groundwork to attempt subsequent prosecution for mental illness, disability or substance abuse pending a psychiatric evaluation.

For severity of abuse to girl siblings of eight years old in the family – 300(j):

"The child's sibling THELMA GOMES has been abused or neglected, as defined in subdivision (a), (b), (d), (e) or (i), and there is a substantial risk that the child will be abused or neglected, as defined in these subdivisions, in that:

(j-1) "In 2007 when the minor Thelma was eight years of age she was sexually abused by her stepfather who also whipped her causing physical injury;

(j-2) "In 2009 when the minor LOU GOMES turned eight years of age she was sexually abused by her stepfather who also whipped her causing physical injury;

(j-3) "On or about November 22nd of this year, the stepfather Mr. Audie Gomes put his hand under his stepdaughter's dress and squeezed her leg, and on December 2nd of this year the minor's stepfather showed her what 'big boys do to big girls' and gave her kisses on her breasts;

(j-4) "There is a substantial risk the minor's sibling AUDREY GOMES, age 7, will be abused, assaulted or neglected after she turns eight years of age, which will occur in a month;

(j-5) "The stepfather has legally adopted Audrey and was made legal guardian of Thelma and Lou in 2004;" and
300(b-1) "The minor's mother Mrs. Cass Gomes has failed to adequately protect her children against the fondling and physical abuse of her husband;" and

300(b-2) "The whereabouts of the biological father are unknown."

The Gomes case was adjudicated on December 4th of this year in Superior Court by Judge Mathew Ellsbe in Department 62. Following Jurisdiction, a finding was made on December 16th of this year for dependency for the minor AUDREY under section 300(j) and for the minors Thelma and Lou for 300(d) and (b) based upon earlier petitions. Stepfather Mr. Gomes was ordered into treatment through Diversion 1000, and to test for substance for fifty-two weeks, he cannot reside in the home of the minors and visitation must be supervised between Mr. Gomes and the minors. The mother was ordered into therapy, and the minors were ordered into art therapy for treatment of anxiety.

Ongoing interviews by the social therapist have resulted in disturbing material. She has conducted six face-to-face sessions of an hour each with the Gomes couple and two joint family interviews and five sessions with just the children. Mrs. Gomes is a very outgoing, friendly custodial parent who nevertheless likes a proper, conservative husband as a father. Mr. Gomes is a strict disciplinarian who believes impurities must be expunged from the body by some form of brandish. His father raised him on the birch, and he feels this is acceptable. He says of the girls they are nice children but 'it's around that age they begin to get a sass and become careless with their belongings forgetting where they put something or just thinking it's okay to give something away.'

The mother Mrs. Cass Gomes says that although Thelma took to Mr. Gomes right away, she didn't want anyone to replace her father. The children's real father left the family when the youngest was two years old and the oldest was four. He had to go overseas on combat and never came back; Mrs. Gomes was told to prepare for the worst. Mr. Gomes came into their lives a year later. She doesn't think Audrey remembers her father clearly; of all the children Audrey tries the hardest to please her stepfather and mother.

When they aren't around their children, they spend a lot of time discussing the news and what Mr. Gomes remembers of his years in the infantry. She says his comments help her in ways to think through her previous marriage. Although this is her second marriage, it is his first. He says that before he met her, he was busy putting his younger brother through college and immediately before that he worked a combat zone hospital as a nurse coordinating medical supplies. As soon as the kids are in high school Mr. Gomes hopes to return to active duty.

The teachers say Thelma is smart for her age, Lou is recalcitrant but can actually quote a person almost entirely, and Audrey is both shy and outgoing. At the moment she has expressed a lot of anxiety over her studies, she has let her grades drop, which is unusual for her, and she has lost assignments which her mother says she has completed nightly.

Analysis: Mrs. Gomes has taken the judge's orders in stride expecting Mr. Gomes shall be allowed to return home soon. The children except for Audrey appear to have adjusted well to their step-dad's absence. The problem of corporal punishment has taken on various implications; Mrs. Gomes doesn't see much difference in her two husbands. Both are military army. Both had similar world views. From the perspective of the older girls this dad has a big problem their dad didn't have, but to Audrey who hasn't known any other dad, the breakup of the home has caused her disruption that his inappropriate touching also caused.

For numerous substances, cocaine, gas, and heroin topper – 300(f):

"On or about February 1, 2010 the minor STEVEN GUNDERSON, age 7, was detained after he was found to be visiting unsupervised in the home of his father, Martin Gunderson, who was convicted in 1991 for causing the death of his first child by an accidental overdose determined to be in the child's food.

"On or about February 1, 2010 the police tested the father Martin for suspicion of drug intoxication as a result of him having slurred speech, he was stumbling, he could not count to ten and the home was littered with gas pellets. The test results were positive for burn cocaine, gas inhalant and heroin trace mixed with cocaine and sugared milk powder.

"On or about February 1, 2010 the police brought the minor to a physician who tested the minor and determined he had ingested cocaine and trace topper sufficient to have caused mild hallucination, and kept the minor under observation in the hospital for three days releasing him only to a nurse foster parent approved by Social Services.

"On or about January 30, 2010 the mother Eugenia Gunderson dropped off the minor to his father because she made plans to leave town for the weekend."

A hearing on the petition was commenced on February 2, 2010 during which the detaining police officer gave evidence. Jurisdiction was found and ordered. On February 12, 2010 the judge ordered the minor Steven be made a dependent under 300(f) and ordered parental rights be terminated. A contest was set by mother's attorney.

Analysis: The minor is age seven and therefore too old to also come under section 300(e) which reads: "The minor is under the age of five and has suffered ... any single act of abuse which causes physical trauma of sufficient severity that, if left untreated, would cause permanent physical disfigurement, permanent physical disability, or death."

The Specialized Treatment Objectives

Social welfare practice varies from state to state and county to county depending upon the size of population served. In California today there are some counties where it is possible for the agency to provide a portion of therapeutic service delivery. In other larger counties where the size of the community served prohibits an agency from providing actual service implementation, the use of modalities may in part or in whole provided to the family unit either in conjunction with various contractual services depending upon the nature of the disposition. In many states including New York, service delivery is entirely incorporated into the relationship the social work professional has with the family.

Each of the four major types of abuse – alcoholism, molestation, physical abuse, and domestic brutality – are discussed for pertinent family dynamics, behavioral constructs and combative issues which may influence the course of treatment. When the social worker meets with the parents, with parents and child, and with the child for face-to-face visits, the social worker must draw on discussions which facilitate an enhanced understanding by each parent as to previous debilitating behaviors either expressed to or acted upon the child. These discussions are points of reference depending upon the family's presenting problem.

Alcoholism

For family identification, rules and roles aimed at warding off anxiety in the alcoholic and essential issues of trust, intimacy and control define the substance abusing family in crisis by their pertinent issues.

* The family-of-origin chaos
* Double messages
* Who was driving the car? or what was in the brown paper bag?
* Fight as a communication style
* Emotional hunger
* Shutting down and stuffing one's creative energy
* The false self - how unique do I have to be?

Rules and roles that helped the family know its limits and boundaries are created by:

* Stages of complicity with each parent
* Behavioral indicators of displacement
* Function of anger, control, all or none reactions, impulse decision making, resistance to authority, fear of loss of self, fear of being found inadequate, fear of closeness and images of abuse and violence.

And core issues:

* Trust and intimacy - how do these occur anyway?
* Learning to breathe; somatic illnesses and what these

reflect
* Identifying body armour and feelings
* Learning to stop being manipulative - methodologies for making the shift
* Endings - what is the hidden fear

Objectives of therapy:

* Tolerate ambiguity without shields of body armour
* Connect actual responses to situations
* Learn to be ambivalent
* Accept one's control is only over one's own decisions
* Extend decision making

Molestation

Treatment for sex abuse is begun in a group sub model, followed by individual insight therapy after about a year, and consists of discussions about secrecy. Unlike alcoholism which is usually obvious and has at least one family identified patient as well as one or more family members around whom a locus of control centers, the family with molest has secrets, which are many times unknown until the victim leaves home. Thus the treatment consists of a modality that looks at behaviors and issues that potentially lead to a revelation of a molesting adult. At that point the victim must be out of the home. If the molesting adult leaves and has no further contact, the child can return home. Thus the modal presentation may consist of these behaviors:

* Bulemia
* Hoarding
* Promiscuity and prostitution
* Drug use
* Teen runaway

The treatment focus discusses:

* Inappropriate touching, skin to skin rubbing, digital penetration, oral sex, anal penetration
* Spouse parent knowledge
* Arranged custodial care or visitation by the assigned caretaker to the molesting adult
* Allowance of a younger sibling to take the victim's place
* Control by the molesting adult over the victim through being the adult who transports, purchases clothing and underwear, forces victim to watch skin flicks with them

> * Control over eating
> * Nudity
> * Bathing
> * Photographs
> * Physical abuse
> * Ritual abuse or torture

The process for the patient of learning to keep his or her physical and emotional boundaries separate from the molesting adult necessarily draws upon accepted practices for child rearing in the home. These include as part of the social work therapeutic treatment milieu for the parents:

* TV to be watched only in a family living room
* Separate bedrooms for different sex children, no shared bathrooms
* Parents to sleep in their own bedroom
* Child's bedroom not to be used for adult guest while child lives at home
* Locks on bedroom doors
* No drugs or alcohol use in the home
* Non offending parent to provide education as to birth control at appropriate age
* Molesting adult never to be in home alone with victim
* No special diets
* No suggestive endearments to victim or other language allowed

* No corporal punishment
* Molesting adult to be in treatment under a psychiatrist knowledgable about the abuse

Physical abuse

In families in which physical abuse is prevalent there is a typically held belief that the child is a psychological extension of the abusing parent. When the abusing parent is overwhelmed or dictated by intolerance that parent can often be found in courts having to address allegations of harrassment, unwanted deprivation and sadism that speaks to real personality disorders. Behaviors of disgust visited upon the child must be addressed both by the social work professional and a psychologist concurrently.

The issues to be addressed by the parents are as follows:

* Physical expediency of anger
* Any behavior that is sadistic in nature, continual hair brushing that includes battery, shoving a spoon in a child's throat, making a child smear his feces, whipping a young teen until they have bloodied welts
* Intolerance with the child's age appropriate developmental state ie age 2 untoilet trained, age 3 making a mess, age 4 wandering off, age 5 losing his coat everywhere

A pathological need to be cruel may be associated with:

* Tendencies to perceive the child is in the way of a promising partner
* An inability to work in a legal marketplace
* A profound, usually understated, hatred of the child

Treatment for the affected minor child is usually permanent removal from the abusing parent when the abuse is severe. In mild and moderate circumstances in which there have been domestic violence episodes the recommended treatment course includes:

* Rehabilitation from drugs and/or alcohol
* Parenting classes, basic and advanced for a minimum of 8 hours each
* Therapy with a goal to psychologically accept and tolerate the child's behaviors
* Gradually increased visitation, initially supervised leading to eventual inhome trial period of no less than 90 days
* Clearance of any criminal charges

Domestic Brutality

In home domestic violence occurs between spouses as a result of escalating arguments often with one or both parents under the influence of a controlled or uncontrolled substance. Fighting often consists of hitting, smashing glass, punching one's fist through walls, biting, destroying objects. Criminal convictions may be sought.

The issue of cohabitation becomes a necessary focus when without a spouse or partner there is an absence of escalation. Children raised in this environment bitterly complain of uncharted aggression in which no person is safe from physicality or violence in the home. Glasses getting smashed, plates being thrown, an adult slamming a person into a wall are examples of violence some adults commit when they are too drunk or too upset to keep their impulsivity in check.

The sole standard must be - is it physically safe to be in the home?

Treatment modalities vary almost none at all. In order for treatment to commence the adult must:

* File a police report

* Press charges against the abuser
* Put the child in a safe place to which the abuser has no knowledge and no access
* Enter a rehabilitation center
* Enter psychotherapy for a minimum of a year

The repetitive problem is the abused adult often returns to reside with the person who assaulted them, despite lengthy separations and an initial phase of recovery. Fundamental ground rules are governed by:

* Agreement to leave before an argument escalates
* Learning how to recognize a disagreement has begun
* Couples counseling for communication skills
* Individual therapy for self management to avoid escalation
* Having names of people to leave to when an argument is out of control

Modality Treatment

Groups for the above problems run a minimum of a year. They meet weekly for six months. Two hours per session is sufficient. Each group not a family should have a maximum of six group participants. Fees for each session range from $25 to $60 per individual and are to be assessed in advance and paid before the group begins.

Each session should have as its basic structure:

* Check ins as to purpose or goal for that session
* Any problems or problem escalations that may have occurred during that week, or information as to the problem that has led them to therapy, 5 minutes each person
* You as group leader may want to assign each week's discussion such as family upbringing, when the addiction started chronologically, key issues, one each week, control, patterns of behavior, dating, longterm relationships,

feelings of insecurity, zoning out, jobs and climbing the ladder, anger, formation of friendships, etc. Each session requires a truthful sharing of each person's personal story
* Notebook work - was it difficult, easy, challenging, insightful etc.
* Check-outs: 5 minutes per person about feelings that came up for you

Dos and don'ts
* Try to search your heart for material anyone shares that you feel you resonate with
* Acknowledge when someone says something that is hard for you to hear and why
* Do not attack another person
* Do not monopolize any discussion
* Try not to fix others by giving advice

Notebook Work / Issues of Focus
Have each group participant purchase a notepad.
Each treatment month is described by open-ended discussion which should become the objective for treatment in discussions both with the social worker and therapists for parents and also for the child.

First month
* Describe what the police report or petitionable allegations reads; discuss in your own language what occurred
* State your rationale at the time of the incident to explain why you were involved; if your partner, child, or other person was there explain what they did
* Talk about any regrets you may have right now; explain also what actions were taken that will affect the future; discuss any legal limitations imposed or to be imposed on you as a result of the warrant
* Discuss who stands out in your life as an angry person and in what ways you think they have affected you

Second month
* Describe your upbringing: where you were raised, who raised you, events both positive and negative to your life under age 21, who you went to for problems, extended family
* Talk about your first dating experiences
* Discuss any youth experiences with the law
* Any insights you've had since you began

Third month
* Any trauma you may have experienced in your life and your reactions to it
* Discuss what feelings you internalized over this trauma
* Describe what you say to people closest to you about feelings: to your partner, best friend, parent
* Make a list of your feelings you have this week and we will discuss them when I come out next

Fourth month
* Describe attributes about your partner and characteristics he/she thinks about you
* Discuss personal pet peeves and communication style, and state what you don't share
* Talk about your ideals and what aspects of your relationship you think you control
* What do you do with negative or unwanted feelings?

Fifth month
* Describe the parenting course you took, what was said about normal child development, typical problems for your age child, what you learned
* Discuss what you think your child(ren) felt because of what occurred — don't ask them, pretend you are the victim and say what you think they now think, what gets in the way of your empathy
* Write a letter to your child and begin with what you think they feel about you in a first paragraph of five or more sentences, admit in your second paragraph everything

you did without making it sensational, and finish with a last paragraph with what you are doing to change and where you are at with that progress

Such a letter must speak to intent, physical injury and psychological assessment, describing behaviors the child is already cognizant of which were they sufficiently changed or eradicated would regain the parent's earned trustworthiness.

"Dear Linda, When you were last at home you heard me scream at your mother. You came downstairs in time to see me punch my hand into the wall. I was drunk and having another blackout. I didn't stop when I saw you which I should have done immediately. Instead I let her have it slugging her in the face and breaking her nose. I was having a tantrum and was behaving like a child. My actions put her in the hospital. I have since served four months in prison for this. I am now on what is called diversion. It is a rehab program for people who get violent. I have stopped drinking. Your mother has stopped using drugs. I am getting better. I take classes and see a doctor. I have to prove to her that I want to be your dad again."

* Discuss last week's exercise and discussion and what came up for you during the week

Hereafter sessions are infrequent yet monthly. Focus is on identifying a support network in the community, obtaining a sponsor, and attending some type of educational program that will put your parents in the open minded psychological state of learning for long enough to change rigid thinking patterns. Material for group discussion needs to center upon an ongoing process of identifying responses to situations. Sessions should explore a consistent set of issues.

Control
Jealousy
Anger
Evasion
Letting Go

In keeping their journals (for each category of issue) you may write events that occurred during the week and feeling states, past typical reactions and negative self talk, such as This week when I went to parenting class the person ahead of me yelled at me during class because I provoked an argument. I felt invisible as if the person was disrespecting me. In the past I would have put my fist in their head. I would have internalized my own self talk, telling myself, "you are about to get beaten up, buddy."

In a journal or notebook the parent with the problems should be encouraged to make every effort to write down what they think they feel in response to situations involving physicality. Typically people who resort to violence feel an emotion or series of emotions before they strike. Often the way they respond is learned over many years by having watched a parent. Thus when the client does his journal writing the only useful tools for recovery involve feeling states to help them begin to accurately connect escalation to actual feeling states.

For control issues: I heard my wife vomit her meal in the bathroom and I wanted to kick her guts in. I found my mother dead in her bed one morning after I'd heard her throwing up the night before when my dad went out to the bar. I had that same old feeling come over me. I felt helpless, like what am I going to do if she (my wife) keeps doing this. It used to be I'd see myself in slow motion. Now I just don't take that 2nd drink.

I don't like arguments. I always lose. There's no one to take my side. Whenever he raises his voice at me when he wants to just out vote me at the yelling polls I pick up an object and let it crash on the floor. That stops him right away. He just walks out. I don't really give a hoot if he's gone for nights. I'm no good at setting my own limits when I've had too much closeness and need my own space for awhile. I've found if I make someone mad they won't come back for awhile. I wind up feeling claustrophobic so much so I can't contain myself. If I could leave, I would. I'd be the first one out the door.

For jealousy: She spends all her free time at his house. If I don't pop in she'd be there all night. Once she stormed out crying and I had to ask myself what's he going to do for her now? I feel cut out of the picture like the way the marriage should be isn't there. I always feel I'm waiting for her to leave me.

For anger: I disconnect automatically when I become angry. I used to see my father break every object of my mother's in the house. When I bought my first car, I'd think that all I needed to do was wait until he slept it off before I escaped. I was usually thinking what he was doing wasn't me, I was numb until I took off in my car.

For evasion: I never tell anyone the real story. When they ask I just tell them what they want to hear. That seems to take care of most problems. It's when I say what I think they want and the person starts needling me over it, it's time to get up and go. Usually I don't feel much of anything. All I'm here for is to put a roof over them, put food on the table. They don't like it, then who needs them. I'm my own person.

For letting go: Letting go of any strong emotion that has taken over one's life requires not acting on a situation that provocatively might evoke anger. This is hard work for individuals who have years of stifling their emotions. They need to build up a new backlog to relearn old familiar destructive patterns.

Behavioral outcomes

Rate of aggression as in frequency has to decline. Without any prevalence of an impulsivity disorder, sheer brutality is considered a risk of detriment in families with minors because when domestic violence gets out of hand it often imposes infliction of wayward violence on a subject too young to not get adversely affected; having thus said, the incidence of aggression, infrequent or otherwise, continues to pose a practical risk for injury. In order for aggression to become translated into other realities, the give-and-take of emotional handicapping has to decline." In discussions with perpetrators the unsavory view expressed is that "a little DV is frowned upon;" their inability to regard their own behaviors as incongruent or an infringement on another's personal rights becomes the goal for therapeutic discernment.

Emphasis is entirely on producing a different mode of thinking such that the responses of the past do not lead to violent or aggressive behavior. In line with this family members need to be encouraged to put all decision making on hold such that it becomes possible for them to sit with discomfort, intolerance, ambivalence and uncertainty. This is the only status that allows them to interrupt their own tendency to act impulsively. By this stage of therapy each member will have had numerous occasions to sit uncomfortably to wrestle with annoyances, a desire to give advice, a tendency to monopolize or seek attention, or any other impulsive behavior.

Expressing Anger In a Healthy Way

- you have to recognize it in yourself when it occurs
- you must be willing to risk changing yourself and in line with this be able to rewrite their own errors in thinking such as utilizing physical coersion
- you must be capable of agreeing to ground rules
- you have to do your own work
- you must teach yourself a new lineup of behaviors to draw on when angry
- you must be willing to share your gut sob stories
- you have to recognize when you zone out and be contientious of another person asking you to zone back in
- you have to be willing to either write or draw during some discussions in order to tap subconscious material

Milestones for change that demonstrate stages of insight

Reaffirm the parent goals,check toassess if the parents have evaluated past interactions.

Test resistance, patience, obstinance, dominance, ie state, as so and so said this, what went through your mind as she was talking.

Do the roles change month to month, is your group open minded or protectively shut down, does the group as a whole take risks.

What do people find difficult to tolerate, are some stories more conducive than others to elicit feedback, during silences does your spouse blame you for not providing commentary or education, have you gently introduced them to an idea that silences are acceptable, are there people who generally don't say much.

You have to decide in advance how your group likes to interact in order to ask questions that will generate responses by many, never pin any individual to a question, don't point out behaviors, don't ask questions that can be answered by yes or no.

- what were people's responses to hearing X talk about feeling a loss of control
- how did people reflect on the admission of evasion
- what makes it difficult when you enter a room full of strangers
- when is it alright to tell a person you do not want to become dependent on them emotionally
- how many entered relationships only to do the awful thing you had promised yourself you wouldn't do like having a baby
- what were you all told about anger and having control over it
- how often did you try to calm an angry person down

This process of looking at high points of feeling thwarted by a strong emotion like anger gradually brings about tolerance, help them to make decisions that are far reaching over many months if not years consisting of but not limited to uncertainty as to choices they will make, structuring home activities, encouraging discussion over dinner, and dividing a parent's time for each child. In addition these adults may have to set limits they have previously avoided.

Letting go - The Second Treatment Objective

The ability to let go offers a replacement value for taking the place of a shadow self which has been controlled by binge drinking, excessive drug use and hiding when neglect points to abdication by the central attachment figure. Letting go of experiences over which the patient has no control is the singlemost objective for treatment. Practically speaking there are many mechanisms which when consistently utilized allow a freedom from the concerns that others are bothered by. These include writing the problem in a journal by date and then permitting oneself to forget about it and returning in several days or weeks to review the need for a decision. Another mechanism is to pass on all decisions as a matter of recourse. Some things must be acted upon: paying bills when one's check arrives, going to the doctor, feeding the dog, providing meals at certain times, going to work, getting together with friends, etc. Aside from these routine mundane responsibilities there is little we need to do.

In the therapy group setting or family the desire to fix someone else rears its head as a continual temptation. Haven't we been in that exact situation and now hearing it from another individual, we know precisely what worked well for ourself. Support is always desirable as long as no one is lectured. Experiences can be shared, each person discussing how they attacked that particular matter.

The modality however, unlike for anger, is brief, about six weeks and ought to begin at around the fifth to sixth month. Some concerns will be new, others will have already been hashed over a great deal.

Limit setting, this concept is essential for without it the individual cannot start to understand that others have personal inalienable rights. The central question each person has to answer for himself is which part of the situation was he involved with. The limit speaks to the recognition that others have participated before and after the event. The corresponding issues may be conceptualized by these following questions:

- Whose baggage is it anyways?
- Will I get what I want?
- Is a decision to act within my control?
- Will I ever be able to say no?
- What helpful aids can I utilize such that I can delay decisions?

The family, if adults, should be able to provide information as to the situation which has led to the court's involvement in their lives. This is the original situation for which a finding has been made as to dependency. In a neglect case the adults will describe their thinking as they allowed the neglect to continue, in an abandonment situation they will describe how the decision was reached, in an emotional count they should be able to discuss how they berated their child, debased him or otherwise harassed him. The sustained counts are written as a petitionable allegation and discussed in a disposition report that provides the evidence of the case. The adult may state, and go on. Then they should be able to clearly identify their journey while in the group, information they have learned, how they have used this information to make changes in their life and the effect it has had on their altering outmoded patterns of behavior. The group can thus ask questions.

Co-dependency, in all abusive and neglectful situations there is a spousal dyad, unless the adult from whom the minor was removed and placed was without a current partner. When the risk of detriment occurred, the adult was doing something to cause it. The questions each adult should speak to are as follows:

- How was parenting done for each task, getting the child off to school, checking over homework, meals, appointments, inviting friends to outings, weekend activities

and chores.
- Who makes decisions pertaining to the child?
- When the child is upset who comforts?
- When the minor loses a possession, what is the adult's attitude?
- What happened at the child's last birthday?

The parents should be able to discuss these questions in retrospect demonstrating a clear view of their attitude and behavior at the crisis and which group discussions most facilitated their changing their reluctance to make a commitment to place their child's needs and concerns before their own. The group/family definition took months and was gradual. They will have identified central issues along the way. Ask them to discuss their process as it occurred to them the type of parent they wanted to aspire to.

Betrayal, as is typical for child abuse court cases at least the non offending parent feels she has been betrayed, if only because she feels were it not for her partner she would not be in the situation. The offender, usually a male adult, feels caught, exposed because his behaviors, previously zealously guarded, are paraded across court papers and he may be sentenced to a prison stay lasting for a year. Emotions may include anger, defensiveness, upset that she has put up with being battered and didn't tell, fear she will lose her husband and won't be able to support herself.

- How often has the adult gone through this?
- Did the adult suffer memories?
- Did the adult talk to another adult after these abuses?
- Did the adult go into a shelter?
- What was the outcome of diversion or treatment?

Trust, at the core of every dilemma either parent or minor child has to wrestle with. In most situations having to come to terms with the abuse already renders the individual to low amount of trust. This sense - that people cannot be trusted and that one's immediate surroundings are not reliably assurred for safety - becomes instilled in the body often as body armour causing the person to retract in situations which others may not view with foreboding. "I cannot fully disclose how I feel" or "I will behave as minimally as possible so as not to make myself the center of attention and get brutalized" stem from a continual exposure to repeated violation of personal rights for a long time.

- When can I stop over reacting?
- How much information do I need to know first about anyone?
- Can I tell a friend about an experience without having them talk about it behind my back?
- Am I a person who trusts blindly?
- How can I reserve my judgement until I have information I would like?

Control, a larger concern is - do they believe they actually can assert control over another person to get them to behave in a way that is more to their liking? Shifting from an idea that this is possible to obtaining information to make informed decisions becomes a focus for being able to let go of obsessive preoccupations.

- Who has power in the situation?
- Can I leave?
- What are the critical issues in this situation?
- What do I think will occur if I do nothing?

The issues of hypervigilance, guardedness and evasion are meant to shield a person against re-exposure to threat. As a set of apprehensive self protection they also prevent spontaneity, trust and assertion. Whereas their behavior may seem aloof or unknowable, there is a certain emotional distance that appears to most people as containment or poise. The real answer then becomes whether the person can cope with their stress and have satisfying relationships.

Letting go, takes years to master. The AA and Alanon groups actively propagate this concept with an affirmation that tells them every time they say it that they are helpless to control the behaviors of others. Asking to be granted serenity is the best one can come to. Letting go is a spiritual act that one derives personal acceptance from. It can form a basis of relaxation for a person not to worry how someone will take care of their own problems. Active listening becomes possible, as does a sense of personal liberation from morbid dependence.

Narcissism

In the treatment of the narcissistic adolescent who manifests hostility the subject grouping of adolescents is two hundred, 80% from broken homes, of which hostile narcissist males represents 32%, many who by age 20 remain in profile characterologically disturbed. These young males predominantly display excessive drinking, gambling, fighting and are quarrelsome, antagonistic and exhibitionist in their interpersonal relationships, behaviors which if left unchecked continue into adulthood in an indulgent demanding mode.

On the subject of hostile narcissism a working definition is a display of malice or hatred to another by someone who perceives their acts will be met with opposition. Dr. Hervey Cleckly, author of The Mask of Sanity, 1976, St. Louis, The C.V. Mosby Co., posits that the individual who chooses crime is a character disordered narcissist who has a personality defect characterized by an inability to feel guilt. He lists a criterion consisting in part a lack of remorse, poor judgement, egocentricity, unresponsiveness in interpersonal relationships, and an impersonal sex life. Hostility is defined as an aggressive act, often a malicious grudge, venomous spite, having a strong dislike to the point of bearing malice. The more severe sociopaths show themselves as bullies, as antagonistic and belligerent, often without restraint, inconsiderate as to what they are putting others through.

In therapy a hostile narcissist is usually a male who has molested, chronically thwarted their victims by bullying, who in their parental authority displays meanness, often times resorting to brutality or violent chauvinism, or a spouse whose cycle of domestic violence involves coercion so as to forcibly draw a recapitulation from the partner. Dr. Sigmund Freud used the term narcissism to describe someone who was so self-absorbed that healthy transference between therapist and patient could not develop. In The *Clinical Handbook of Marital Therapy*, edited by Neil S. Jacobson and Alan S. Gurman, (New York: Guilford, 1986) chapter consultant Dr. Melvin R. Lansky of Department of Psychiatry, UCLA Medical Center, Los Angeles, says of narcissist males they are "self centered, needy of attention seeking admiration, humiliation-prone viewing others as extensions of self," "narcissistic injured and narcissist vulnerable, their parents being emotionally absent; they have feelings of being incomplete, cheated," engage in wrist slashing, binge drinking, overdosing, competitive gambling; in spousal relationships "they are people who need each other to hold each other together to avoid exposure of personal defects" such as feeling empty, or without awareness and competency of a core personality. While this collusive relationship in adult life may prevent relational disasters, their state is nevertheless seen as "developmental arrest." Therapy that cannot facilitate differentiation must begin with "the patient's turbulence," considering how shame occurs in the patient when he feels defective, damaged such that he believes himself to be unable to control his destructive urges. Likewise an inability to shore up positive regard for oneself is described by David H. Olson, PhD, Amy Olson-Sigg, and Peter J. Larson, PhD, in their notebook *The Couple Checkup* to take the form of negative put-downs, negative focus, and prejudice, thus making breaking out of domestic escalation difficult and exploring role-incongruent behaviors almost impossible.

Conduct disorders not included, the syndrome appears to be cyclonical, creating its own chaotic intra-personal disorganization. Dr. William S. Sahakian, ed., *Psychopathology Today*, 3rd edition, F. E. Peacock, Inc. borrows from the American Psychiatric Association, from Diagnostic and statistical manual of mental disorders, 3rd ed., Washington, DC: APA, 1980, for compulsive personality disorder – an individual with "restricted ability to express warm feelings for others, perfectionism that interferes with an ability to see the big picture, an insistence" through marked behavior "that others submit to their way of doing things, excessive devotion to" legal or illegal "work, stinginess with emotions, preoccupation with rules, efficiency, and trivial data, and relationships of a dominance-submission dynamic." A narcissist personality disorder gives an individual whose focus of behavior manifests "grandiose preoccupation with unlimited success, an exhibitionist need for constant admiration, interpersonal exploitation, lack of empathy, ambition that cannot be satisfied," a fragile ego, with chronic devaluation of others. William McCord and Joan McCord define the psychopath as "an asocial, aggressive, highly impulsive person who feels little or no guilt and is unable to form lasting bonds of affection."

Sahakian refers to Dr. Hervey Cleckley's use of anxiety ratings, specifically the Taylor score and MMPI score, to derive a diagnostic criterion which includes "an absence of neurotic anxiety, irresponsibility, inability to distinguish between truth and falsehood, and an inability to accept blame." Sahakian further notes from P. Greenacre, 1945, that present in the psychopath lies "a faulty structural development of the conscience" in which the described character defect is acts based upon impulsivity rather than as a result to being overwhelmed by pressure.

In my own study of adolescent mothers who are chronically hostile to infants, 90% who by age six would batter or brutalize a younger sibling, utilizing a grouping of 25 mothers, the demonstrated problems were: refusal to teach sons to urinate by age six (11), chronically placing a diaper over the baby's face (6), and not holding the baby and also not making eye contact (6). Little has been written on the subject of maternal hostility as a precursor to hostile narcissism in males of pre-adolescence or adolescence. Weakland, 1960, and Craft, 1965, in discussions as to etiology believe the severity of disturbance in the child is owing to an adverse parental relationship. This adversity is neither resultant from loss of the maternal figure as Bowlby cites in children who mourn their mother's death, nor from a double-bind communication typified by schizophrenia. The hostile mother rejects her role altogether; not wanting a child to begin with, they nevertheless do not agree to place the infant for adoption. In these youngsters soothing does not occur but coincides with feeding; mastery of milestones such as crawling, sitting and climbing becomes postponed in a conflict that engages rage; identification of parent is absent, so is gazing about, pointing, other interests of objects disinclined; the child stares vacuously; failure to bond is noticeably absent.

Conscience does not form where attachment is absent. The mother/child dyad is the foundation by which reality, control of instinctual aggression, thought processes, defenses, self, and the ability to assimilate the external world into self is organized (Horner, 1984.) The predominance of anger and anxiety over pleasure and relief from distress, wherein rage of frustration, anxiety of uncertainty and lack of basic trust wind up in emotional detachment and passivity (Erickson, 1950.) Mahler, 1971, states that the depriving mother who cannot respond except for basic tasks of dressing and feeding, who is inconsistently available for holding, talking and playing, has caused a disruption of attachment which in turn motivates a defensive detachment when the child eventually loses interest in the parent. Bowlby agrees especially with regard to the task of imprinting, of forming relatedness and a sense of self; early maternal deprivation has a predictable outcome in psychopathology. Horner herself views the maternal role as a mediator of cohesion of self for having a sense as to the rights of others that inadequate attachment manifests in significant distress. Daily social interaction between infant and primary caretaker is the essence of attachment; without proximity-maintaining behavior, Bowlby contends the child is presumed not to achieve object constancy. Klopfer states that a failure of the environment to provide an uninterrupted replacement object through preadolescence will lead to the adult becoming self-centered, prone to transient indiscriminating relationships, and continued separation may elicit intense and violent hatred for the abandoning attachment figure. In the psychopath the more security needs are frustrated, the more the development of ego becomes crippled.

Because we had a prevalence of sexual hostility cases I tried to look at personality elements that might produce better definitions. Men with hostility in situations of sexual aggression fall into two categories - dangerous and exhibitionist. It is the dangerous perpetrators for whom criminal activity renders them in a mask of neurotic indifference that their experience as males is defended. In order to penetrate this mask, to get the subject to be willing to risk exposure of self, the therapist has to confront the comfort that danger consists of, without devaluing the confidence that masculinity can provide. Tolson, 1977, speaks of "conflicts, jealousies and reconciliations" which in many men are characterized by "ambivalence and an analytic barrier." Complex self-definition involves a social definition of work and family life; Tolson says further that "the power of men is the social language of which man is the subject. Built into masculinity itself there are three main points of stress – the relationship of the married couple, relations between parents and children, and the experience of sexuality itself." The implications for the contradictions are to be found in the devaluation of children by men through violence, in the 60/40 split of pay, lack of childcare and lack of advancement.

Appendixes

First Interview With Parents – Suggested Format for Parent's Ability to Protect

— Do you agree with the police narrative?
— Do you believe the court report accurately describes the incident?
— Can you tell me what occurred?
— Was this the first time?
— How did you respond?
— Are you seeing a therapist, or are you in a program?
— What have you discussed?

I have met with your child. He is polite and well-mannered. You have raised him well. From now on I will meet him several times a month and with you and your partner once to twice a month or more frequently if additional support is indicated. During each visit I will ask for information from you about your personal upbringing, form of discipline you have used, progress you are making on your Case Plan and your perceptions about the usefulness of the services you have received. The information you provide is expected to be consistent with what happened. When I have to submit my summary in a report to the court every six months I will review it first with you.

In this report under Progress Made, you must address the criteria as to genuine empathy for the child. Is empathy operative? Is the severity of the incident viewed with accuracy? In your assessment you ought to be able to state that the parent demonstrates sensitivity to the child's need for protection or the parent lacks empathy and cannot protect. Other questions are: is the custodial parent able to nurture emotionally; and did this person take the child's side or did this person justify the abuser's behavior?

On family of origin, the first interview for this consideration should include the following questions,

—Did any parent have a problem?
— In what ways were they abusive?
— What did they say about it?
— How did the other parent manage?
— With siblings, was there competition for attention from your parents?
— Did anyone in the family have secrets?

For each working parent,

— For how many years have you held down a paid job?
— What are the pressures of the job?
— Does your spouse or family approve of the type of work you do?
— Do you have outside family obligations?
—When do you have contact with the abuser?
— Does the child's father attempt to alienate him from you?

Commonly Asked Questions

What makes a person normal?
　　The predictive range for normalcy comes about with several factors analogous to human behaviors. These include an ability to express warm feelings, be empathic, tolerate ambivalence, acknowledge differences of opinion; cry, actively listen with acceptance to another person; demonstrate abstract thinking, be able to be non-violent, relatively non aggressive; and possess an ability to learn. Two psychiatrists developed summaries about an individual's inability to preserve honest transparent emotion states. Richard Bourne, 1978, stated that without therapeutic intervention minor injuries to a child were likely to become major consequences, and severity of response increases over time. Melvin Lansky, Department of Psychiatry, UCLA, 1981, states any kind of injuries – physical, sexual or traumatic – to a child causes emotional absence, feeling of being incomplete, binge drinking, wrist slashing, overdosing, being humiliation-prone. Loss of identity cues create an absence of psychological safety. In Koretsky's study, 2004 out of twenty-five children under the age of five who battered other younger children, six were not taught to urinate.

The DSM-IV describes Reactive Attachment Disorder as developmentally inappropriate social relating that begins before age 5 years. In the Inhibited Type the child persistently fails to initiate and respond to most social interactions in a developmentally appropriate way evidenced by a pattern of hyper vigilance, excessively inhibited or high degree of ambivalence with frozen watchfulness. In the Disinhibited Type there is a pattern of diffuse attachments owing to a persistent disregard of the child's basic emotional needs for comfort, stimulation and nurturing; or repeated changes of primary caregiver that prevent formation of stable attachments.

According to Diane Harkins, MSW, Packard Children's Hospital, Stanford, 1995, the task of childhood is to regulate affect. The task of late adolescence and adulthood is to regulate emotions. Maltreated children react strongly and quickly, use fewer expressive words, take fewer opportunities to explore their environment, and demonstrate less complex play. These character disordered children increase aggression when their victim cries; however, when their victim is hurt, they verbally attack, incapable of displaying soothing nurturance. Of these trait disordered youngsters, 65% are from neglected homes; they show failures in meeting emotional developmental milestones and are wary in trust, loss, guilt, control and identity. However, the psychological effects of mistreatment for interrupted development, failure-to-thrive syndrome, the parentified child and acting out behavior and disturbances of mood derive from sexual abuse or physical abuse. Physical injury generates the highest control issues of any of the personality traits and disorders.

In "The Cycle of Bonding: Interruptions from Abuse and Neglect," in *Understanding and Treating the Severely Disturbed Child,* by Foster W. Cline, M.D., Evergreen, CO., 1979, Cline contends that the child who does not experience a predictable cycle of nurturing later displays an inability to grasp an outcome relationship causality of cause and effect and has no conscience. The first eighteen to thirty-six months are critical because a baby who has suffered disruptive contact from a culture of impermanence develops a heightened sensitivity and irritability that leads him to have problems learning role relational reciprocity and emotional development.

Out of this upbringing the resulting adult can be characterized by strong pervasive feelings of sadness, despair or failure, feelings of being unloved and guilty, difficulty dealing with angry feeling states, inability to make decisions, slowed thought processes and sleep disturbance. Nihart, RN, Turning Point Center, San Francisco, and Veterans Administration Medical Center, Menlo Park, describes when the self becomes the target of aggression, the person adopts inescapable destructive traits and weakens their defense mechanisms by splitting, projective identification and devaluation.

As to life transitions author Charlotte Eliopoulos, MPH, (*Gerontological Nursing*, 2010) in assigning contributing factors to nursing diagnoses says, "One of the hallmarks of successful …" transition of life phases "is knowledge of self – that is, an awareness of the realities of who one is and one's place in the world. From infancy on, we engage in dynamic experiences that mold the unique individual's we are." The repetitive acts of challenging one's sense of the world, indeed of having apprised life goals and outcomes from time to time restores a finite proof as to "what drives them to behave as they do, or what their true purposes and pleasures are."

When discussing how adults learn to overcome trauma, one must necessarily draw upon the realm of psychology and its allied treatment in order to comprehend the need for personal change. Psychology is the study of non anatomical motivation into our own behavior and stresses we encounter in daily living. It is the practice of sitting down to discuss with guided assistance what we believe and experience about aspects of life and living. In the social work setting the task of therapy is to increase health for the family who has stopped functioning with psychological safety. Thus, the goals of psychotherapy consist of the psychological exploration of delving into oneself to create a release from stress, suffering, and maladaptation. Goals can include insight into what one thinks and instructs oneself about events in one's experience, freeing oneself from an internal critic. As therapy unfolds, this exploration facilitates the grouping of experiences into a collection of symbols and truths.

C.G. Jung wrote in *Analytical Psychology: Its Theory and Practice* that the seeking individual relies upon the active imagination in order to make the unconscious able to be understood and dreams and writings about images and feeling-values inherent in symbols of dreams as ways to work through a non supportive parent wherein the patient had internalized a negative self-image and was afraid he was right that he was bad. Jung harnessed the powerful release that the patient who displays an overly developed intellectual expression of experience by valuing his emotions through a drama of speaking to them in dreams. In addition, working out images through writing about them, or through drawing or painting, the patient can investigate his or her Self scientifically, thus arousing their own intuition and fascination. By working out intricate problems, one may see into them without fear of censure for a positive effect that is tangible.

In *Civilization and its Discontents* Sigmund Freud discusses the purpose of human life in terms of what a person wants to achieve. He says the goals of life are an absence of pain and unpleasure and to derive an understanding that happiness – the satisfaction of needs – as "an episodic phenomenon." Suffering can come from the body, from the external world, and from relationships to others. Goals tend to be contradictory such as an unrestricted satisfaction of every need, avoidance of unpleasure may push obtaining pleasure into the background, voluntary isolation, happiness of quietness, become a member of a community working for good. Freud advises that to shore up against reality without self-numbing through intoxication and withdrawal from pressure of reality, one should base satisfaction of instinctual drives as opposed to "killing off instincts with undeniable diminution in the potentialities of enjoyment." This latter reality can lead to alienation. The goal is to increase yields of pleasure from psychic and intellectual sources. The artist's joy in creating or the scientist's solving problems prevent displacement of instinctual objectives. Independent of the external world the life of imagination helps a person be receptive to art and combat against depression and withdrawal from vital needs.

Joseph Campbell in *An Open Life*, [Perennial Library, New

York, 1989], established that the purpose of one's life is to create metaphor for the Self so as to broaden one's outlook. "Myth is metaphor." Dreams are metaphoric of structures in the psyche; art interprets the inner life in terms of relevance of experience. Campbell describes the essence of structuring one's life for meaning – there is "The Call," or visionary quest, and the Hero, the one who reports on the quest. He says, "Through your own inward experience, awe of life is found. Myth takes a person through stages of a lifetime."

How do people lose track of their lives?

For many, there are circumstances which the individual tolerates out of endurance but which offer very little pleasure or interest. If this dissatisfaction lasts for several years, the subject may display apathetic mood, suffer from moderate depression and in general feel fatigued and empty, like nothing is worth the bother or worn out in exerting energy.

The crucial concern is to determine how to get from – What should I do in life? – to, What is Meaningful?

Divorce, I am told, takes forty years. After a serious crisis, one erects a protective buffer around the Self – life is separate, out there somewhere. When nothing comes to mind except empty feelings, start with an image, a drawing, for example of your yard. Sit down with a dictionary and select words to put later into a paragraph of creative reflection about your illustration.

> vititate
> wane
> plight
> nourish
> tranquil
> redemption
> clemency
> forthcoming
> trumpet
> abstinence

Maurice Nicoll in *Dream Psychology*, [Samuel Weiser, Inc, NY, 1979] introduced myth in the dream that arises from somewhere out of the psyche. Myth-making collection leads one inevitably to psychical investigation. A patient tries to push problems out into a shadowy part, not fully aware as to how it manifests. The welling up of energy permits ghosts to unpredictably put a strain on one's waking life. These tensions are viewed as exhausting as if there is an internal barrier that is stymied.

"The ability to feel or hear the intelligence of your body and its memories is a very important survival skill." This excerpt of Jennifer James, author, *Visions from the Heart*, describe what she terms knowing intuition for aspects of living or being that are otherwise invisible or unknown, that exist in thoughts from experiences in the past or within the world. It is the frantic pace of life, becoming overwhelmed and unable to cope that prevents the individual from fully participating in life with meaning. James discusses solitude and patience of waiting for recuperation from illness.

Parental compliance, what are basic tasks?

The essential tasks for compliance rest with successful completion of the court-ordered case plan. In almost all reports the case plan contains four or five criterion which often involves weekly psychotherapy, a eight hour parenting class taught by a parent educator, drug or substance abuse testing, and regular appointments with the assigned social worker. The parent or parents must be able to demonstrate during the course of treatment that they understand the allegations in terms of their behavior and be seeking constructive ways of addressing and changing whatever was deemed a risk of detriment to their child or children. It is not enough to simply go through the case plan activities; they have to show that they understand the risk and that they are gaining insight into their own motivations and ease of parenting guidance.

What is foster care?

Foster care is an alternate home setting for the child who is adjudicated a dependent child in the Welfare and Insititutions Code 300. Such care may include actual homes operated by a trained, licensed foster parent; a group home in which counselors work six-hour shifts; a special program for a teen mother and baby; or a facility where the school is situated on the premises such as a dual-diagnosis house. The duty of the foster parent is to provide a safe house, three meals a day, educational support, transportation to school, after-school activities or therapy, and some type of stimulation such as baseball games, Little League, music lessons or academic tutoring.

When is an IEP conducted?

An IEP is an Individual Education Plan usually created specifically by the Unified School District for the child who is behind or delayed, or conversely for the gifted child with an above-average Intelligence Quota. The parent or foster parent or guardian must request an IEP thirty days after the child is enrolled. The school district then must by law test for aptitude within forty-five days of the request. Eight categories are tested. These are English composition, spelling, language construction, intelligence quota, self-expression, and science efficiency. Once the categories are rated a report is prepared. The Vice Principal with one or more teachers and a district psychologist meet with the social worker to discuss primarily whether the current school is the appropriate academic placement for the child. At these discussions the school may approve special education hours or a behavioral modification school setting for the fire starter or aggressive student.

When is a toddler recommended to a school for special services?

By the age of three, a toddler who lacks basic skills will have been referred for special education hours along with his mother or primary custodial parent. Most counties have a specialized daycare or Wee Care school. These are set up with several large rooms, adaptive toys, and are staffed by two nurses trained in infant and toddler stimulation. Reasons for referral are inability of the child to pay attention or to focus, combative aggression in interactive play, thwarted hostility or rage, and frustration turned inward.

In which child abuse situations does a natural parent experience resurging guilt?

The most typical situation is the one in which there has been a molestation by either a natural relative, including a natural father, grandfather, uncle or brother, or by a stepfather or family friend, including but not limited to a minister or family physician. The non-offending spouse often perceives the situation as something either actually within their control, or that they should have established control of activities inside the home. This may have been watching television in a bedroom, using an only bathroom while a teen was showering, or the molesting incident may have been a much greater manipulative incident such as a family member waiting until the mother left to go to work. Because the treatment necessarily depends upon the parent trying to determine where they were when the abuse occurred, it is not uncommon for that parent to become bogged down in a particular time period.

Why is it important to obtain a police report?

A police report is taken at the time of the incident. It gives a narrative summary that defines what happened and who acted upon the victim. It is commonly provided for domestic violence when the victim of a beating or a neighbor overhearing an out of control fight calls 911. As a tool for witness evidence, it usually provides a unbiased account and may be helpful in court to establish the facts for an injury or threat. The social worker should discuss the report with the offender and spouse during the first interview and second if deemed necessary in order to assess each parent's willingness to agree on what occurred.

What does outpatient rehabilitation consist of?

Usually outpatient treatment is provided for inability to stay sober and may involve family violence. The parent in treatment attends three groups a week, receives individual therapy, substance abuse tests, and has supervised visits with their child. Groups look at abuse, daily use patterns and relearning interactional skills. Individual therapy explores personal issues, often family of origin work, domestic violence and/or family violence, medicating oneself, injury such as cutting one's wrists and relationships. Most outpatient programs occur at night after the parent gets off work.

What can a parent do to provide family cohesion?

The most noteworthy problem of a substance abusing parent is their failure to provide a safe environment with a strong interactive family identity. In order to instill a child with positive values, the parent has to be a role model. The best manner to establish positive self-esteem is to have family sit-down dinners nightly over a prepared meal put onto plates with silverware. Over dinner the parent should talk about how their day went, ask their spouse what they did that day, and let each child five years or older say something. The information should be friendly. More serious talks should occur away from the child's presence and cannot become major disagreements with slapping or other violent acts. In addition to eating dinner together every evening, the parent may join a church, take their child to church for baptisms and confirmations, and develop a support group through an Alcoholics Anonymous at church or attend picnics.

How does the law view a step-parent?

The Welfare and Institutions Code states only biological parents of a minor child are entitled to receive a Case Plan. A step-parent does not have any privileges in the eyes of the Court. However, a parent who has legally adopted or who became legal guardian does. In implementation of the Case Plan, the natural parent has to ensure that the step-parent follows the law. The custodial parent has to assure physical as well as psychological safety to the child; the child cannot be beaten or molested; the natutral parent has to make certain the step-parent does not bring perpetrators to the home, does not get drunk or use drugs and lose control over their own behavior. The natural parent must demonstrate that they are able to protect the child first over and above the needs of the step-parent.

When is a paternity test ordered by the Court?

If there is a question as to who the parent is or are, the Court may order all parties or the parent in question to take this test. For paternity to be proved, there must be a test on file for the minor or the minor also has to surrender a blood test. This testing is usually handled through the County Clerk, requires an appointment, and takes about three weeks to receive results.

What essential aspect must give way just prior to insight in order for the aggressor to accept resolution?

The point is reached when the abuser is willing to recognize that he or she has caused the problem that existed for the child. Often just reaching this point is an uphill struggle lasting a year or more. Many offenders are not interested in setting the facts straight and want to offset the pressure they perceive by having others feel sorry for them. The answer is a slow answer – there will be no way for the family to predict when they are willing to become flexible.

Under what set of circumstances is it considered normalcy to have to request a disturbance be treated asymptomatically?

There can be no overriding transference projected by the subject. This lack of animosity must be maintained for over eight months. If acted-upon hostility tests for validity, every effort needs to be made to determine whom the diagnosed patient has targeted. If testing reveals ambivalence without a hostile target the patient may be said to be asymptomatic. An inability to keep thoughts within the latitude of ambivalence suggests that the disturbance is again manifest.

Animosity is reinforced when the patient requires the defensive shield in order to collaborate in secrecy some aspect of past living he does not want to become known. Whether the defensive shield is due to ill feeling such as acrimony or animus, or crosses a boundary of intent and is in fact malevolence has to be the determinant for symptomatic behavior at which point duty to warn has to be evaluated.

Criterion might be –
* Verbal assault without provocation
* Combativeness
* Intent to incite or instigate so as to leave result of primordial insult by injury
* Wanting to produce an atypical reaction from the therapist
* There is no one person who is the source of agitation, this agitation is generalized

In what situation or situations might it be conducive to test for paranoid trait when treating a narcissist?

Narcissists position content of descriptions for memory that is meant in their mind to last eternally. Most people change their idea of what has happened over time, but these people hold to a rigid fixed belief. The narcissist usually perceives he is held by others in a beneficial light, and there is no sense he has hurt another, even if he has. "The child is always waiting for me before he makes me upset." "In her house I'm at fault." "She's always critical of me." Here, there is a clear belief system operative that there is another person the patient views has a negative consequence on him, but the paranoia trait does not hold to his concern for long.

The narcissist has no complaint. The world revolves around him because he has capabilities. (His view) There is no sense of the world not viewing him with high idealization. A narcissist with paranoia trait now has a complaint, there is someone who is contrary to him and in that person's view he is devalued. Since it would be healthy if the narcissist were depressed, seeing perhaps for a first time that they may have been hurtful, one would have to include additional criteria: domestic violence, using illegal drugs or alcohol dependence, or demonstrates increasing hyper vigilance or to a lesser trait degree displays Obsessive Compulsive Disorder.

When should a borderline be thought of as narcissistic?

When the person has become suicidal – it is with a typified borderline whose defensive behavior is to view no consolidation of self as having made a resolution when that conflict appears over.

What is the rationale for the protocol on teen runaways?

Girls run, boys drink is the proverbial saying about teens who find their home life too intolerable to deal with. The majority of teen runaways are females between the ages of fourteen and seventeen. They usually run to the home of a non custodial parent out of a need to experience family connection especially after an argument with a custodial parent or group home counselor when sharp feelings of loss and remorse are perceived. The desire for a more lenient home environment often influences their decision – a place to hang out without the pressure of personal responsibility. It is not unusual for a runaway to be addicted to drugs.
After age sixteen many county jurisdictions will not actively issue a warrant on a runaway unless the teen surfaces as a participant in a crime or is found to be homeless. In nearly every situation in which a teen placed out of the family-of-origin home makes a direct beeline to their family, they believe their mother has permitted a molester into a home where sibling children are residing. If the police have cause to believe a teen intends to commit a murder, they may issue a warrant, but in today's world even if the teen has left behind a suicidal note, the police will not attempt to search for a missing teen to apprehend her or him until the minor has been missing 72 hours. Because addiction and drug-induced emotional numbness can lead a teen to a house where methamphetamine is manufactured and used, the runaway may be tracked over county and interstate lines, thus necessitating an arrest warrant. A runaway will be hospitalized in a sanitarium under a 5150 only if she or he is displaying active homicidal or suicidal ideation and then arrangements are made for placement in a hospital locked ward or in a dual-diagnosis foster home supervised twenty-four hours by therapists.

What is going on with rage release?

Rage occurs where the teen cannot adequately protect against an inability to cope. This state may take years to build up to or may occur suddenly and without warning. When out-of-control rage does occur, the teen has already anesthetized emotions, constricted obvious usual responses, and is attempting to control thwarted needs through denial, particularly through a sensate barrier that insulates Life, keeping it psychologically safe from illusion, boredom and grief. Loss of control over behavior signifies a departure from fitting in with society, becoming increasingly withdrawn, morbidly so, or conversely becoming increasingly anti-social, inept at skills that were high functioning, unable to be restorative in handling crisis and eventually handling day-to-day considerations.

What function does motivation play in behavioral crises?

Motivation is the spit and glue that cements an individual's reasonableness over pressures of living. In itself it constitutes the ways in which responses to events are conceptualized. In the circumstance of rage, motivation becomes quintessential in determining whether the individual's repertoire of normal behaviors gives him clarity of optimum functioning, choices with which to test ground, ability to recognize when to solicit help and above all, a clear-thinking approach to utilize numerous avenues of response to deal with problems as well as with happiness. With overly subjective manipulative motivation, fallacy of thinking is operative and loss over control becomes dominant. Motivation has to be assessed when this loss seems imminent especially if the individual can respond to treatment within a less restrictive setting. An MMPI and a Rorschach should be given as minimum baseline tests in conjunction with any other series of question ranges and evaluation interviews.

The child in a state of trauma is locked in by fear. He or she is often unable to have a sense of what the problems may have become. This state is like a soldier who has fought in a war on the enemy lines whose battalion has been plundered and other men have lost limbs. Soldiers who return are often still panicking; they have interiorized an experience of sudden death, overwhelming brutality, and have cut off emotion from truth, sequestering that valued part of their responsiveness behind confusion or drunkenness or drug abuse.

What lab tests reveal extent of neuro-psycho-chemical addiction?

Testing should be commenced as soon as intoxication becomes observable such as slurred speech, stumbling gait, extreme shakiness, foul breath, belligerence, hard breathing or loss of consciousness.

Standard substance abuse testing consists of urine testing done in the presence of a public health nurse usually through a health department or a private lab. This test should evaluate the urine for the presence of alcohol, cocaine, crack cocaine, amphetamine, methamphetamine, heroin, and/or marijuana, at a minimum. The number of grams are reported per substance determined, with a low of 10 mg. designating trace and 200+ mg. representing a high amount of saturation. Additional testing for overuse of pharmaceutical drugs should also be given, when possible, such as for Valium or Xanax or a street drug MDMA known as Ecstacy. In situations in which a person is in treatment with the use of Valium, the individual must be under the care of a licensed physician.

How might a child learn to self-soothe?

For the child the early beginnings to replace listlessness or inattentiveness or illness may be to draw or paint. Color enhances a child's awareness. By their curious nature they gravitate to bright colors. These are a delight and comfort for a child who seeks to self-soothe, amuse and create stimulation. With the advent of touching toys, color becomes a natural compliment to activity; it elicits attention … splashing colors together, draw, release tension and become personally content.

In that psychology is the study of non anatomical motivation into behavior and stress, in social work it is the treatment of families who have stopped functioning in a healthy way that places a child at risk or in detriment. The goals of psycho-therapy have at the locus of a psychological exploration of delving into oneself the task to create a release from the perception of trauma. The child relies upon active imagination in order to make perceptions and emotions able to be understood utilizing symbols and representations and to value their emotions speaking to them in dreams. Working out images through painting, the young person can investigate the Self scientifically, thus arousing their own intuition and fascination without fear of censure, producing a positive effect that is tangible. An essential goal in living is to increase pleasure from intellectual sources; in an artistic milieu it is the joy of creating; for a science-minded individual it is solving problems. The life of the imagination helps a person be receptive to art and guard against withdrawal from vital needs. It depends upon how much restraint, frustration or pent-up energy the child displays, but generally two one-hour sessions a month for six months is recommended. As a child grows older the ability to comprehend the needs of the psyche and its memories becomes important to creating positive self-definition. The child who can learn to utilize intuition for aspects of his personality that are otherwise invisible or unlearned that exist in thoughts from experience of the past or in the world helps him to create solitude and comparison.

"Myth is metaphor," said historian Joseph Campbell, 1989. Art interprets the inner life of a seeking person. Through an individual's own inward experience, Campbell stated that an awe of life is found. Myth provides a belief in what is meaningful.
For many who have suffered some form of loss or trauma, the internal emotional state develops a buffer around the Self until life seems separate, out there somewhere. No inspiration comes – for the child the initial beginnings to shrug off this armor is to start with a drawing. Color is very important to the awareness of the child. By their curious nature they gravitate to bright colors. These are a delight and a comfort for a child who seeks to self-soothe, amuse and create stimulation. With the advent of touching toys, color becomes a natural complement to activity; it elicits attention and focus, without which a young child left to

their own carefree or casual spatial capability with no adult input becomes quiet, non interested or bored. The sudden, energetic release by finger painting or drawing takes on a great deal more sophistication for the use of gooey bright, fast-drying paints. A few squirts onto the medium lead a normal child to playfully create, splashing colors together, draw, relax and become personably content.

For the therapist the task of painting can be evaluative. A complying child who does not protest or rebel but who remains mild mannered has an ability to be lulled into a relatively calm state especially after a group exercise involving expenditure of pent-up constraint. On the other hand a school-age defiant minor who disobeys, demonstrates difficulty behaving with deference and passiveness, or who stirs up or strikes out may be subdued by the introduction of color. Not as remedying as television which departs stimulus from a child's self-defeating regimen, color nevertheless recategorizes insurgent energy into calm non-resistance.

Limitation by no means implies harness although an older minor in their teenage years might try to break loose with such art as cubism, impressionistic representation, or incorporate as yet unlearned skill into an essentially restrictive discipline. Despite this perception, I recommend acquiescence to release, a focus almost entirely upon color rather than form, a fun disposal of inquiry. Indulging the child in whatever drawing or art that answers their sense of restraint, frustration, or entreaty may take two one-hour sessions a month for several months; however, ought not to occur at all to discover unwilling inhibition which may signify coping stress and serious interior deterioration.

As a child grows older "the ability to feel or hear the intelligence of the body and its memories" becomes a very important survival skill. (Jennifer James, Ph.D., 1991) Utilizing intuition for aspects of the personality that are otherwise invisible or unknown that exist in thoughts from experiences in the past or within the world helps create solitude and patience. "I said to my soul, be still," James quotes T.S. Eliot; creating a visitation to the psyche facilitates a psychical investigation, conscious or otherwise, when a youth tries to escape problems before being fully aware as to how the problem manifests. The attempt to dam up a reservoir of stifling energy keeps a child detained from their essence through doubts, negative self image, contradictory feeling states, impotence, and so on.

Similar to adults who are displaced by virtue of having escaped a war-torn country, many children experience the trauma of having been raised in an embittered antagonistic or hostile environment wherein they were viewed as secondary to the relationship between the spouses or as keenly non compensatory without adequate enrichment that most families thrive on. The tests on endurance for the war-depressed adult surrenders him to a sense that the world is plunged into a dormant, sometimes chaotic life over which he receives generous to adequate support but from time to time is set adrift in an unpredictable tide. For the little guy who finds himself poorly equipped to meet the demands of these tests of patience, the need to quickly assume strengths that will defend him becomes convincingly assured.

Charts

These statistics are not a study. They represent a total of 2,150 spouses and 820 children seen in clinical interviews over a ten year period within office, private and public sectors. Comparisons are based upon nature of presenting problem.

Of 2150 parents and 701 children seen for interviews between 1991 including through 2000, approximately 340 were family groupings which required family systems therapy of viewing the family members together as well as separately. Severity consisted of: at least 2 parents both alcoholic; 1 parent bulimic mother; sex abuse almost all men narcissists. Each parent set was deemed high risk when the following conditions were met: mother unipolar, father bipolar, step-father abusive. Of single parent families the criteria for highest risk was abandonment. 85% of separated families reunited in a year to eighteen months after problems were exculpated – teen depression requiring four-day hospitalization most noticeable at early stage of divorce; primary parent admitted with one to two children under age seven, one a newborn; and failure to thrive infants due to parental neglect who required two week hospitalization with physician orders as to feeding alone. Overall high risk education together with paid employment of at least one parent, joined by spouse for couple systems counseling kept a child in good health the longest. Dynamics necessitating initiation of intensive interviews were children held at risk when family was not intact. Need of child to be with mother outweighed all risks.

As to the efficacy of the model, what worked in the interview that produced positive outcome was a careful organization and structuring of questions especially as to family of origin, improvements in communication so as to feel listened to and use of support networks. Additionally having the social worker model transparency; set limits; discuss the abusive behavior and secret-keeping, what the child experienced and what the parent thought; and report on therapy and groups – did parent apply learned skill during the week, lowered anxiety and freed the parent to experiment with interactions. Outcomes included decreased risk, increased tolerance, sincere empathy and bond attachment.

What didn't work with process of interviews included monitoring progress without discussion of change of family dynamic; discussion of allegations without a police report lacking a way to hold parent to accountability; and failure to use police for safety checks as to who parent allowed to stay in the home at night and on weekends.

Parents	2150
Single	590
Couple	1650
Adjudicated	1009
Children	701
Normal	637
Delayed	64
Abuse	701
Physical	50
Neglect	422
Emotional	140
Sibling	59
Abandonment	30

Number children who are returned

Year	# Rem	# Ret'd
1991	30	25
1992	45	28
1993	45	29
1994	50	35
1995	50	40
1996	40	30
1997	60	40
1998	45	25
1999	50	41
2000	50	46

Number of alcoholics who do not recover

1991	16
1992	18
1993	21
1994	18
1995	20
1996	25
1997	19
1998	24
1999	20
2000	15

Appendix: Charts

Number of mothers who are unsympathetic	
1991	12
1992	7
1993	30
1994	15
1995	12
1996	10
1997	25
1998	14
1999	16
2000	19

Number interviews for parent implementation		
1991	40	780
1992	70	480
1993	90	1350
1994	90	880
1995	105	1132
1996	140	1410
1997	122	1310
1998	107	1120
1999	73	961
2000	92	1061

BASIC CURRICULUM

The basic curriculum for clinical child therapy licensees focuses on both intrapsychic and systems approaches. It looks at the healthy family including the system in crisis. Discussion gives expression to the transparent self as well as introductory material on transference, counter transference, and personality. However it does not lead to a psychologist license. Most who take child and family coursework will acquire toward an MFC license.

Standard coursework requires knowledge in:

1. Counseling theory
2. Research
3. Statistics
4. Group procedure
5. Relationship
6. Family therapy
7. Law & Ethics
8. Psycho-Pathology
9. Internship

Thus the training for the family and child practitioner includes:

- MFC
- MFT
- CSW
- Early Childhood
- Addiction
- Interns

Apprendix: Charts

# Blended interviews/ Molest/Emotional trauma for children			
1991	12	.60	.90
1992	38	.30	.75
1993	40	.50	.50
1994	20	1.00	.50
1995	10	1.00	.80
1996	22	.70	.25
1997	30	.70	.90
1998	15	.90	.90
1999	20	.60	.75
2000	30	.50	.50

# Blended family interviews and % blended seen for therapy		
1991	12	.01
1992	38	.05
1993	40	.10
1994	20	.50
1995	10	.00
1996	22	.20
1997	30	.25
1998	15	.60
1999	20	.50
2000	24	.08

Number domestic violence and injured children			
1991	40	8	.75
1992	70	11	.90
1993	90	16	.80
1994	90	12	.95
1995	105	20	.60
1996	150	37	.68
1997	130	40	.73
1998	107	32	.56
1999	50	10	.95
2000	85	17	.80

* Level of opportunity is great.

Suggested Reading

Basic Job Skills Training Child Welfare Services: Trainees Coursebook "Diagnosing Severity of Physical Abuse as a Case Management Tool," 1987 by Bowdry, Carole W., MSWW, Texas Department of Human Resources Protective Services for Children.

The Disowned Self, Branden M.D., Nathaniel; Bantam Books, New York, 1972.

Challenges of Humanistic Psychology, Bugental Phd, James F.T., McGraw-Hill Book Co., New York, 1967. Articles by Maslow, Abraham, Wyatt, Frederick.

Personality Development and Psychopathology, Cameron, Norman, p. 640.

The Observing Self, Deikman M.D., Arthur J. Beacon Press, Boston, 1982, pp. 4, 5, 13.

Greatness and Limitations of Freud's Thought, Fromm PhD, Erich, New American Library, New York, 1980.

The Nature of the Child, Kagan PhD, Jerome; Basic Books Inc., New York, 1984. pp. 240-276.

The Politics of the Family, Laing M.D., Ronald David, Vintage Books, New York, 1972.

The Dynamic Family, Luthman LCSW, Shirley Gehrke, and Kirschenbaum PhD., Martin; Science and Behavior Books, Palo Alto, CA 1974.

The Search for the Real Self, Masterson M.D., James F., pp. 54-58.

Intimate Behavior, Morris, Desmond, Bantam, New York, 1972.

Crisis Intervention: Selected Readings, Parad, Howard J., Family Service Association of America, New York, 1965. "Short-Term Family Therapy," Mordecai Kaffman. "Children at Risk," Elizabeth E. Irvine; reprinted from *Case Conference*, Vol. 10, No. 10, 1964. "A Unit for Mothers and Babies in a Psychiatric Hospital," from *Journal of Child Psychology and Psychiatry*, Vol. III, No. 1, 1962. "Multiple Impact Therapy," Agnes Ritchie, reprinted from *Social Work*, Vol. 5, No. 3, 1960. "The State of Crisis: Some Theoretical Considerations," Lydia Rapoport, from *The Social Service Review*, Vol. 36, No. 2, 1962. University of Chicago Press.

Love and Addiction, Peele PhD, Stanton, Signet, New American Library, New York, 1975.

Healing The Child Within, Whitfield M.D., Charles L., Health Communication, Inc., Deerfield Beach, Florida, 1979.

Science, Feb. 2008, "Learning with Regret," by Cohen, Michael D., School of Information, University of Michigan, Ann Arbor.

Science, Oct. 2007. "Decision-Making Dysfunctions in Psychiatry — Altered Homeostatic Processing?" by Paulus, Martin P.,

Department of Psychiatry, University of California at San Diego, and Veteran Affairs Health Care System at San Diego.

Smart Marriages Institute, 2008, The Coalition for Marriage, Family and Couples Education, San Francisco CA, "Love Without Hurt" by Stosney, PhD, Steven; "The Couples Checklist," by Dr. Olson, Donald.

Attachment and Rage

APA. *Diagnostic and statistical manual of mental disorders.*, 3rd ed Washington: APA, 1980.

Bowlby, J. "Grief and mourning in infancy and early childhood" in *Psychoanalytic study of the child,* Vol. 15, 1960.

Bowlby, J. *Attachment and loss in Loss, sadness and depression.* New York: Basic Books, 1980.

Cleckley, H., *The mask of sanity,* St. Louis: C.V. Mosby Co., 1976.

Craft, J., *Ten studies into psychopathic personalities.* Bristol: John Wright, 1965.

Doroff, D., "Developing and maintaining the therapeutic alliance with the narcissistic personality." In *Journal of American Academy of Psychoanalysis* 4, 1976.

Greenacre, P., "Conscience in the psychopath," in *American Journal of Orthopsychiatry,* Vol. 15, 1945.

Greenacre, P., Ed. *Affective disorders.* New York: International Universities Press, 1965.

Greenson, R., "Disidentifying from mother: its special importance for the boy." In *Explorations in psychoanalysis.* New York: International Universities Press, 1968.

Horner, A., "Stages and processes in the development of early object relations and their associated pathologies," in *International review of psycho-analysis,* 1975.

Horner, A., *Object relations and the developing ego in therapy.* New York: Jason Aronson, 1984.

Jacobson, N. and Gurman, A., *A clinical handbook of marital therapy.* New York: Guilford, 1986.

Jacobson, E., *The self and the object world.* New York: International Universities Press, 1964.

Kaplan, Helen Singer, *The new sex therapy.* New York: Times Books, 1974.

Kernberg, O., *Object relations theory and clinical psychoanalysis.* New York: Jason Aronson, 1976.

Klopfer, B., *Developments in the Rorschach technique*, Vol. II, Yonkers on the hudson: World Book Co.

Kohut, H., "Thoughts on narcissism and narcissistic rage" in *Psychoanalytic study of the child,* 1972.

Lansky, M. R., Department of Psychiatry, UCLA Medicine, Los Angeles, 1986.

Lichtenberg, J.D., "The development of the sense of self." In *Journal of American Psychoanalytic Association,* 1975.

Mahler, M.S., Pine, F. and Bergman, A. , *The psychological birth of the human infant.* New York: Basic Books, 1975.

May, R. *Power and innocence: a search for sources of violence.* New York: Dell, 1976.

Olson, D. H., Olson-Sigg, A. and Larson, P., *The couple checkup.* Nashville: Thomas, 2008.

Rogers, C. R., *Client-centered therapy: its current practice, implications and theory.* Boston: Houghton-Mifflin, 1951.

Rutter, M. "Maternal deprivation reconsidered" in *Annual progress in child psychiatry and child development,* eds. S. Chess and A. Thomas, New York: Jason Aronson, 1973.

Sahakian, W., ed.., *psychopathology today.* third edition. Ithaca: Peacock, 1986.

Satir, V. *Conjoint family therapy: a guide to theory and technique.* Palo Alto: Science and Behavior Books, 1967.

Siegman, A. D., "The relationship between future time perspective, time estimation and impulse control in a group of young offenders and a control group." *Journal of consulting psychologists,* Vol. 25, 1961.

Spitz, R., *The first year of life.* New York: International Universities Press, 1965.

Sutherland, E.H. and Cressey, D.R., *Principles of criminology,* 6th ed. Philadelphia, Lippincott, 1960.

Weakland, J., "The double-bind hypothesis and 3-party interaction" New York: Basic Books, 1960.

Zuk, G. H. and Boszormenyi-Nagy, I., Eds., *Family therapy and disturbed families.* Palo Alto: Science and Behavior Books, 1967.

On Masculinity

Berne, Eric MD, *What do you say after you say hello?* New York: Grove Press, 1972, for chapters on "Parental programming."

Faraday, Ann, *Dream power.* London: Pan Books Ltd., 1956.

Greene, L., *Relating.* York Beach: Samuel Weiser, Inc., 1978, for chapter "Beauty and the Beast."

Johnson, R., He, *understanding masculine psychology.* New York: Harper, 1989.

Krishnamurti, J., *Commentaries on living*, 2nd Series, Wheaton, Ill.: Quest Books, 1968.

McCord, W. and McCord, J., "The psychopath: an essay on the criminal mind" in W. Sahakian, ed., *Psychopathology Today*, 1980.

Lowen, A., *Fear of life.* New York: McMillan, 1980.

Stein, M., ed. *Jungian Analysis.* Boston: New Science Library, 1984, for "Treatment of children" by E. Sullwold, MFC.

Tolson, A., *The limits of masculinity.* New York: Colophon Books, 1977.

On The Law

Edwards, Leonard P., Hon., *West's California juvenile laws and court rules.* Los Angeles: West, 1992.

Symposiums

Young, Jonathan, 2002, "Psychology of Creativity" and 'The search for meaning." San Diego.

Carnes, F. MD, 2003, "On narcissism." Los Angeles.

Young, Jonathan, 2004, "On mythmaking" and "The beloved of the soul." Los Angeles.

Smart marriages, Family and Couples Education, 2007, 11th Annual conference, Denver. John Gray, "Mars and Venus Collide;" Harville Kendrix and Helen LaKelly Hunt, 'Imago Connects,' Howard Markham and Marcie Pregulman, "The future of marriage," Steven Stosny, "You don't have to take it anymore," and Barry McCarthy on "Rekindling desire."

Weisner, Stan, 2007, UC Berkeley, "Understanding and treating anxiety disorders."

Smart marriages, 2008, 12th Annual Conference, San Francisco. Stevn Stosny, "Love without hurt bootcamp," David Olson and Mathew Turvey, "Prepare/Enrich," Frank Pittman MD, "At the movies: Raisin in the sun, Heartbreak kid, Mr. and Mrs. Bridge, Rambling Rose, and Network," and Bob Ruthazer, "Bootcamp for new dads."

www.ingramcontent.com/pod-product-compliance
Lightning Source LLC
Chambersburg PA
CBHW030318080526
44584CB00012B/609